ACKNOWLEDGMENTS

To the millions of family caregivers who make unimaginable personal sacrifices to foster the well-being of seniors in need. You are the heroes who give all that you have to ensure your aging loved ones continue to thrive in the face of life's most difficult hours.

TABLE OF CONTENTS

The Handbook of
Live-in Care

A Guide for Caregivers

Kathy N. Johnson, PhD, CMC

James H. Johnson, PhD

Lily Sarafan, MS

The information contained in this book is intended to provide helpful and informative material on the subject addressed. It is not intended to serve as a replacement for professional medical advice. Any use of the information in this book is at the reader's discretion. The authors and publisher specifically disclaim any and all liability arising directly or indirectly from the use or application of any information contained in this book. A health care professional should be consulted regarding your specific situation.

 Printed in the United States of America. For information address Home Care Press, 148 Hawthorne Avenue, Palo Alto, CA 94301.

ISBN 978-1-4507-7953-1

ONE
Introduction to Live-in Care

Live-in care encompasses the physical, psychological, social, and spiritual care provided to a person (usually a senior) who is largely or totally confined to their home, wheelchair or bed as a result of age, illness or injury. Thanks to advances in medical care, it is now rare for a person to spend all of his time at home. Most people can occasionally be transported by ambulance, wheelchair van, or private vehicle, if only for medical appointments. However, if a person spends the majority of his or her time confined to the home or an institutional setting, and can leave that setting only with difficulty and with the assistance of another, he may still be considered in need of live-in care.

What is Live-in Care?
Live-in care is defined as around-the-clock care for a person who cannot be left alone, even for a short period of time. Most live-in care is 24 hours a day, 7 days a week.

Who Needs Live-in Care?
People of any age can require live-in care. However, there are three general conditions that most often result in the need for live-in care.

Temporary Health-Related Conditions
Some people require live-in care temporarily and make full or partial recovery. For example, it is often recommended that people in hospitals have a full-time "sitter" to serve as a companion or even as a go-between with the nursing staff. Other examples

include those who have had a stroke and require live-in care while they go through rehabilitation and relearn the skills necessary to care for themselves. Rona Caburian, Care Coordinator of Home Care Assistance in Palo Alto, California, shares the example of older adults who have had knee and hip replacements. "After their surgery and a stay in rehab, these seniors usually have live-in care for a month or two until they can resume their normal activities. Live-in care helps them transition from a facility to the home, and get back on their feet fast."

Chronic Health-Related Conditions

Chronic conditions remain stable or slowly get worse over time. Examples of chronic conditions include paralysis resulting from a spinal cord injury, Parkinson's disease, or frailty associated with old age. In these cases, live-in care is often seen as preventative measure for people who are at risk for falling or are in need of general support to live alone in their own home.

Terminal Conditions

Terminal conditions are life-threatening illnesses or injuries that are expected to end in death. For most people who are terminally ill, life does not stop and live-in care is often needed, even if only for a short time. Examples of terminal conditions include cancer that has spread throughout the body or advanced Alzheimer's disease. Lena Vyrva, C.N.A., of Home Care Assistance, Palo Alto, California, reports that live-in care can be extremely beneficial for terminal clients. "Live-in caregivers often provide assistance with medications for pain and to control symptoms of nausea or vomiting. Plus the caregiver becomes knowledgeable about all the daily living activities that make life just so much easier. Live-in caregivers also make sure that the individual with a terminal condition is comfortable at all times."

Who Provides Live-in Care?

Live-in care is provided by a wide range of people, ranging from family caregivers, such as spouses or adult children, to professionals —usually Certified Nursing Assistants or Home Health Aides from Home Care agencies. In some cases, the live-in caregiver is a family member who has received little or no formal training and learns about caregiving "on the job." Many of these family caregivers find themselves providing care without any professional assistance or advice. If you are providing live-in care to a loved one, this book is for you.

What Does A Live-in Caregiver Do?

When most people think of providing live-in care, they think of physical care—feeding, bathing, dressing, grooming, toileting and changing bed linens. This book will provide step-by-step instructions on how to complete all of these tasks with a loved one. However, it is important to realize that the needs of a senior are more than just physical needs. This is best illustrated by referring to the work of psychologist Abraham Maslow.

Need Hierarchy

Maslow argued that every person has a "hierarchy" of needs. And once one set of needs is addressed, another set becomes prominent. Maslow's hierarchy is often depicted as a triangle with basic survival needs at the bottom and more abstract emotional and spiritual needs at the top. Maslow believed that to truly thrive, a person must have all of his or her different needs addressed.

Physiological Needs
All of us share the same basic physiological requirements—the need for food, drink, shelter from the elements, sleep, treatment of illnesses and injuries, and so forth. This book will help you become aware of what is needed to meet a person's basic physiological needs.

Security Needs
According to Maslow, once physical survival is assured, most of us turn our attention to security. We want to feel safe and secure in our environment. We don't like feeling as if our world could turn upside down at a moment's notice. Typically, people who have experienced even marginal helplessness due to a sudden illness or injury have difficulty regaining a basic sense of security and trust for the world around them. As a result, an important part of any caregiver's responsibility is making sure that a sense of personal security is established.

Social Needs
Humans are social by nature and dislike feeling isolated or cut off from others. Many seniors experience a shrinking of their social world. While often this is not talked about, it is an extremely important component of caregiving. And it can make a great deal of difference to a senior's happiness. There are many reasons why an older adult may find it difficult to maintain an active social life. Friends may feel uncomfortable visiting. ("I don't know what to say. We don't have anything to talk about any more.") Spouses, friends and other family members may have died. The senior may have difficulties with his hearing. No matter the reason, the end result is that seniors may be left to spend too many hours alone.

Often, a primary caregiver is too busy to address the person's social needs—or doesn't think that these are important. One senior who spent most of his days alone while his son worked explained why he preferred a professional caregiver from a home care agency: "With my agency caregiver, I finally have someone to talk with."

Self-Esteem Needs

As people, we like to feel competent, be knowledgeable and be recognized for what we do well. It is important for each of us to be good at certain things and to be recognized for these abilities.

Simply existing isn't enough. We want more than to just be alive—we want to be valued for our thoughts and our abilities. We have to be doing something or to have sought-after opinions to be considered worthwhile. No matter how old or how chronically ill, we want to be listened to and believed in. This basic need is called "self-esteem" and it is extremely important to well being among older people.

It's not surprising that many people who need live-in care suffer from low self-esteem. Chronic illness and accompanying physical limitations have a way of draining feelings of worthiness and are hard on self-esteem. Grishelda Lancanlale, Care Coordinator, Home Care Assistance of San Francisco, California, remembers one senior who was confined to her home by a particularly painful form of bone cancer. "She would always share sad feelings of 'not being good for anything anymore' with me." Grishelda noted that this woman cheered up considerably when she began live-in care. "The live-in caregiver found out she loved to draw so she helped her paint pictures for each of her 16 grandchildren." As a caregiver, you will need to help your loved ones maintain their self-esteem. This may involve just talking, but more likely, it will involve keeping a positive attitude and working together on a task or project, or even assisting in with volunteer work or a charitable contribution. Maintaining self-esteem is different than other caregiver responsibilities, but it is no less important.

Self-Actualization Needs
Maslow theorized that once all of a person's other needs have been fulfilled, then he or she should focus on "self-actualizing." To Maslow, this involves becoming the very best human being one can possibly be. Maslow estimated that only a small percent of the world's population achieves self-actualization. Among those that do, he identified several common traits. These include: focusing on reality instead of wishful thinking; adopting a problem -solving stance rather than bemoaning life's difficulties; and viewing the journey through life as being just as important as the final destination. The caregiver's attitude can influence a loved one's feelings about the world. Often the caregiver and the person needing live-in care can work together to help each other actualize and get the most out of life.

This book will help you discover ways to address your loved one's care needs. You will also find a chapter devoted to meeting your own needs as you travel this road as a caregiver. Whether you're looking for technical information on giving a bed bath, ways to avoid embarrassment as you provide personal care or tips on how to increase self-esteem, this book will provide help and encouragement.

TWO

The Facts on Live-in Care

No agency throughout North America keeps exact statistics on the number of people who receive live-in care. Some pieces of research, however, hint at the answer.

Characteristics of the Person Receiving Live-in Care

In 2007, the United States Census Bureau revealed that 37.9 million U.S. citizens were over the age of 65. According to the Alliance for Live-in People, one in 20 individuals over the age of 65 is not able to get to doctor's appointments due to a physical or a cognitive disability. Taken together, these figures imply that there may be as many as 1.9 million seniors in the United States who are living alone or with a caregiver.

According to a 2004 study sponsored by the National Alliance for Caregiving (NAC) and the AARP, and funded by the MetLife Foundation, the average age of a person requiring care at home is 75. The most common reason for needing care was listed as ordinary frailty due to aging. Other common diagnoses requiring home care included diabetes, cancer and heart disease.

Dementia is another common reason that seniors may require live-in care. According to the Alzheimer's Association's *2010 Alzheimer's Facts and Figures*, 5.3 million people in the United States have Alzheimer's disease. Of these, over one-third will remain at home through the end of life. The Alzheimer's Association estimates that in 2009, 11 million unpaid caregivers, mostly family and friends, provided 12.5 billion hours of unpaid care. The Alzheimer Society of Canada estimates that 420,600 Canadians over 65 have Alzheimer's disease and related dementias. This means that one in 11 Canadians over the age of 65 currently has Alzheimer's disease or a related dementia. The prevalence of dementia continues to increase throughout the United States and Canada.

A commonly overlooked group of people that may require live-in care consists of younger people. In the 2004 survey of caregivers mentioned above, one in five caregivers reported they were providing care to someone aged 18-49. The majority of these people had short- or long-term physical conditions, such as spinal or head injuries. However, 23% of younger persons requiring live-in care suffered primarily from mental illness, most commonly depression or a developmental disability.

Characteristics of the Caregiver Providing Live-in Care

Just as there are no definitive statistics on individuals with live-in caregivers, there are no reliable statistics on the caregivers that help them. Again, information must be estimated from various research projects and agencies that advocate for caregivers.

One of the most recent studies of caregivers appeared in the Journal of Family Practice in 2009. This study was limited by a small sample size (22), a limited geographical scope (Baltimore, Maryland), and the fact that it included paid caregivers. The average caregiver in this study was 59 years old, Caucasian, female and providing unpaid care to a person with whom she had spent nearly 40 years of her life, usually a spouse or a parent.

The previously cited 2004 study sponsored by the NAC and the AARP was more comprehensive, surveying over 1,200 unpaid caregivers throughout the United States. Because this study defined a caregiver as an adult who helped another adult with at least one or more activities of daily living (ADL), such as eating, toileting, bathing, etc. or instrumental activities of daily living (IADL), such as shopping, caring for pets, or managing money, not all of the caregivers surveyed were providing care to live-in individuals.

The study found that roughly 21% of the entire adult population provides some form of unpaid care to another adult. Of those identified as caregivers, 17% stated that they provided more than 40 hours of care each week, and 31% reported providing the highest level of physical care. In this study, 61% of caregivers were female and 39% were male. The average caregiver was a 46-year-old woman providing at least 20 hours of care a week to her mother. However, 22% of respondents indicated that they provided care for two adults and 8% were responsible for providing care for three or more.

57% of caregivers who provided the highest levels of care had no other employment and over 65% lived with the person requiring care. Most caregivers said that caregiving had little effect on their physical health, although there was a correlation between the level of care required by the older adult and the likelihood of the caregiver to report his or her health as fair or poor. 34% of caregivers said they felt high levels of emotional stress. Younger caregivers tended to report less stress than middle-aged or older caregivers. Those who felt they had no choice in becoming a caregiver were most likely to report higher levels of stress.

The survey also found that becoming a caregiver to a family or friend resulted in less time spent with other loved ones, less time spent in leisure activities and less time spent engaged in healthy practices such as exercising. When asked how they managed stress, caregivers reported several popular coping mechanisms, including prayer (73%), talking to friends (61%) and seeking additional information about caregiving (44%). 27% said they had spoken with a professional or spiritual counselor, and 12% said they had taken or were taking medication for a stress-related condition.

Another helpful coping mechanism was reaching out to the community. Almost half of caregivers reported that they had sought financial assistance, formal training, support groups, or services for their loved one, such as respite care from a non-medical home care agency like Home Care Assistance.

Even with healthy coping styles in place, more than two-thirds of caregivers reported having unmet needs in their life. More than half report a serious level of depression. 82% of people providing 40+ hours per week of care and helping their loved one reported needing additional resources and support.

The Bottom Line

Chances are, if you are caring for an older adult, you are one of the majorities of people who say that they could use additional information and support. This book will help guide you in caring for your loved one while still meeting your own needs.

THREE

The Beginning of Live-in Care

The need for live-in care starts in one of three ways. It can begin as the result of a sudden illness or injury. It can begin as one of many stages in a chronic disease process. Or it can start as the result of frailties developed over the course of a long life. How live-in care begins typically reflects how caregivers are chosen and how they view their responsibilities. The sudden onset of caregiving may also influence how the individual feels about his condition.

Sudden Onset

Sudden onset illnesses or injuries usually involve catastrophic events like head injuries, spinal cord injuries, strokes, or massive heart attacks. In these cases, live-in care does not typically start at the moment of the injury. Instead, the person starts in a hospital to be medically stabilized. From there, the person may go to a rehabilitation facility or a skilled nursing facility. Or, they may also decide that care at home is the best option.

Jill Cabeceiras, Care Manager of Home Care Assistance, Oakland, California, shares the story of her client, Josie. "One day Josie called me and said she wasn't feeling well. Josie has always been totally independent, never wanting any help in her home, so I knew something was wrong. I said I would come to her home to visit. Josie always leaves her garage door open for me when she knows I am coming. This time, however, the garage door was closed. I rang the bell, but no Josie. I called her and although she picked up the phone, she said she couldn't get out of her recliner. Josie also said she felt strange and she did not even remember calling me. I realized something was very wrong and called 911. When the paramedics arrived, they suspected she was having a stroke. To this day, I'm so glad that I was there for her. As the ambulance took Josie to the hospital, I followed and made a phone call to her family. I waited at the hospital until her children arrived. She was diagnosed with a stroke. This fiercely autonomous woman never regained her ability to walk. It all happened so fast. Suddenly she was confined to bed and only able to return home with live-in care."

Before deciding which type of care is most appropriate, it is important to consider a variety of factors. What can the individual do himself? What kind of physical care is required? What kind of cognitive care? Are there any resources for in-home support or medical equipment available?

Families then need to ask themselves some difficult questions. Are there one or more caregivers available—family or professional—who are physically and emotionally able to handle the person's needs? Are the living arrangements in the home limited, or can they be changed to accommodate a live-in caregiver? Are there sufficient financial resources available?

Many families face the reality that they are not equipped to care for their loved one at home by themselves. They need to plan to pay for in-home care provided by a home care agency. This approach can be the best of both worlds. Keeping a person in the comfort of their home has countless benefits, health and otherwise, not to mention a lower risk of infection and falling.

However, there are costs involved that are not covered by Medicare or regular insurance. A special type of insurance called long-term care insurance covers home care.

Peggy's Story

Peggy is a 64-year-old woman who was involved in a serious car crash and was paralyzed from the neck down. Peggy's family consisted of her husband, Frank, who worked full-time. After months in a rehab facility, Frank brought Peggy home. He arranged for neighbors to stay with her while he worked, but they were not always reliable and he sometimes came home to find his paralyzed wife all alone. Eventually, he contacted the local Home Care Assistance office and interviewed several candidates before selecting two trained live-in caregivers to provide the care that he could not. Frank no longer felt guilty, knowing that Peggy was receiving professional care, and he knew that he could spend quality time with her. Peggy and Frank thrived with this care arrangement.

Gradual Onset

Many illnesses progress so slowly that the individual may become home bound almost before the family knows what is happening. If an appropriate family caregiver is not available, families need to consider professional care from a home care agency. If dealing with a terminal illness, a hospice company can provide support for the entire family.

Dwight Wilson, CEO of Mission Hospice in San Mateo, California, recalls the slow progression of one of his clients: "I had both the pleasure and opportunity to watch one man care for his brother of 52 years with pancreatic cancer. Both men had very limited success in navigating through life, financially and personally. Essentially Jake and Ned had each other and not much else. Jake was unemployed and Ned was dying from cancer. Ned had a long history of drug abuse and anger management issues. He was on Medi-Cal and did not have health insurance."

"To look at both of them, one would have to ask the question: how is this going to work as Ned's disease worsens? How could anyone support such a family constitution as Ned slowly loses his ability to care for himself and needs live-in care? Given the limited resources available, how can this situation work?"

"The fear of dying, losing control and having no family did not bode well for success. What Jake and Ned did have going for them was a loving bond that had developed between the two, and a hospice team committed to working with them. If Ned became verbally abusive, the hospice staff gave him room to de-escalate. When Jake's unemployment insurance was close to running out, our hospice social worker assisted in extending it. When certain care issues needed to be addressed, several volunteers were able to be in attendance."

"When all was said and done, Jake was able to help Ned die in his own home. Despite the worst fears by those of us who were caring for the brothers, they somehow made it work. My take away from this experience is never underestimate the power of love and devotion when caregiving for a loved one, even when there are significant challenges that lie ahead in the dying experience."

Jessica's Story

Another option for many families is relocating the older adult to live with an out-of-town family member. For instance, Jessica lived in Austin, Texas. Her mother, who had started to show signs of dementia, lived in Kansas City. Jessica's mother had been born in Kansas City and had many friends who still lived there. She always said that she didn't want to leave. Despite her growing intuition that things were not going well with her mother, Jessica monitored her with nightly phone calls and tried to tell herself that her mother was just a little forgetful.

One night, Jessica was awakened by a call from one of her mother's friends. She had seen Jessica's mother's picture on TV as an unidentified emergency room patient. Jessica called the hospital in question and learned that her mother had wandered out of the house wearing only a bathrobe. When police stopped her over a mile from her home, she was so confused that she could not even tell them her name.

In spite of her mother's initial protests, Jessica brought her mother to live with her in Austin. There have been no more wandering episodes and Jessica reports that her mother, though frail and forgetful, seems content.

Caregivers who take over in a crisis, like Jessica, may find themselves at a disadvantage to caregivers who respond to a sudden-onset illness or injury. This is because they are unlikely to have received any formal training in their new roles. A gradually worsening condition usually does not call for a hospital or rehabilitation center stay, so there is no discharge planner or social worker to arrange for necessary medical equipment or to educate family members.

Finding Help with Caregiving

If you are taking over the role of caregiver for a friend or relative whose condition is worsening gradually, ask your loved one's physician or a local Geriatric Care Manager (www.caremanager.org) about recommending services for your loved one. You may also want to seek training in your community. Both the Red Cross and the Alzheimer's Association, as well as many local senior centers, offer training programs for family caregivers.

Whether the disease process is sudden or gradual, chances are that your loved one will grow tired and frustrated with being at home all the time. The next chapter suggests some activities that you can do together to help stave off boredom and perhaps even help your loved one find a new sense of meaning in life.

FOUR

Activities for Home Bound Seniors

Activities for home bound individuals will vary widely depending on their interests, physical abilities and cognitive abilities. These activities can be for entertainment purposes only, or they can have a utilitarian function, such as caring for oneself or helping the household to run more smoothly. The right activities can help your loved ones meet their social and self-esteem needs. In general, there are three types of activities that caregivers find useful: Passive, energetic and interactive.

Passive Activities

Passive activities require no participation on the part of the senior. Watching the television, listening to the radio, reading and sleeping are all examples of passive activities. Passive activities are not bad—most people enjoy sitting in front of the television for a little while every day or taking an afternoon nap. Furthermore, your loved one may have physical and cognitive impairments that prevent him from participating in active or interactive activities. In that case, leaving the television or radio on is preferable to hours of silence.

If your loved one is more active, however, try to limit passive activities such as watching television to only a few hours a day. And when you do provide passive activities for your loved one, try to make them meaningful. For instance, rather than simply turning the television on to whatever channel happens to be playing, try to find programming they might enjoy.

One woman who was providing care for her home bound (and very confused) mother went to a thrift store and bought her a collection of Little House on the Prairie DVDs. Her mother had enjoyed that program when it first ran years earlier and loved seeing the familiar characters again. Whenever her daughter put on a DVD, she would clap her hands and say excitedly, "The farm show!" Sometimes finding a program your loved one will enjoy means putting your own preferences on hold.

If your loved one is cognitively impaired by Alzheimer's or another form of dementia, avoid crime dramas or violent movies. People with dementia often have trouble with reality testing—distinguishing what is and isn't real. They often think the people on the television set are in the room with them and can become understandably frightened at having a gunfight going on in their bedroom.

Sleeping

If your loved one has a terminal illness, being very tired and spending more and more time asleep can be a natural progression of chronic disease. If their illness is not terminal, however, keep an eye on how much they sleep during the day. If you think they are sleeping too much, have a word with their primary care physician to determine which sleep patterns are normal and which are not. People who are recovering from an illness or injury may genuinely need lots of rest. On the other hand, seniors sometimes sleep a lot because they are bored or depressed. You may need to gently encourage them to become involved in more active or interactive pursuits.

Energetic Activities

These are activities that require some involvement and response from a person. They can range from doing puzzles such as crosswords or Sudoku, drawing pictures and craft projects to getting dressed or helping prepare dinner. Activities that require some action on your loved one's part can be extremely positive for self-esteem.

You can encourage your loved one to be active in many ways. One of the most important contributions you can make is allowing them to do as many activities of daily living as possible. Activities of daily living involve the things we do to keep ourselves alive and healthy—moving around, maintaining personal hygiene, dressing and eating, for instance. Even though a loved one may have physical or mental impairments, and even though it might be quicker to just provide care without their help, offer the chance for participation. Every little bit of independence the person maintains will play a role in increasing self-esteem.

It is also important to continue to participate in instrumental activities of daily living. Instrumental activities of daily living are not necessary for survival, but they do help maintain a sense of choice and independence. Examples include shopping, managing money, caring for pets or plants, preparing meals and doing housework.

Dennis' Story

Dennis had a challenging problem. His father, Hans, owned and operated his own business since he was a young man. Every night before kissing his wife and son and turning out the light, Hans carefully balanced his books. A stroke at the age of 87, however, damaged Hans' eyesight and left him home bound and confused.

There was obviously no way he could remain in control of his business accounts. Dennis, however, didn't have the heart to tell this to his father. Instead, he purchased identical pairs of accounting books. Dennis took over the business and kept the real accounts, but Hans had his own books and painstakingly wrote numbers that made no sense to anyone but himself. This continued until just a few days before he died. In this creative way, Dennis preserved both the business his father had worked so hard to build and his father's dignity and sense of importance. Balancing the books was also an activity that kept Hans happy for hours on end. It was a solution that worked for everyone.

Other instrumental activities of daily living that your loved one may be able to help with include folding laundry, dusting shelves, helping with shopping lists, watering plants, wrapping holiday presents and assisting with caring for pets.

One housekeeping activity that is not usually a good idea is vacuuming. It's just too easy to get one's feet tangled in the cord, which can lead to a nasty fall. If your loved one has cognitive impairments, you should also discourage cooking or ironing unless you are available to closely supervise.

Other activities that require your loved one's participation include reading, writing, drawing, making shapes out of non-toxic clay or Play-Dough, doing jigsaw puzzles, doing crosswords, word search puzzles, or Sudoku, and helping to sort and identify old pictures. Use your imagination. You will be surprised at how much fun you are able to have.

Interactive Activities

Interactive activities are activities that rely on connecting with a person or pet. Sometimes the best activity of all is just having an engaging conversation. You can talk about a news story that interests you, something funny that happened to you at work, or share a favorite childhood memory. You may also just want to sit quietly with your loved one and hold hands or offer a backrub. Time spent in silence with someone you care about can be just as precious as time spent discussing a topic.

Nina Pflumm Herndon, Executive Director of Sage Eldercare Solutions (www.sageeldercare.com), shares this advice in the Handbook of Geriatric Care Management by Cathy Cress:

- Social interactions can be supported by coordinating regular communications from family and friends, such as a once weekly 'telephone date' with a sister in another state or a best friend from childhood.

- Consider a "Presto" printer (www.presto.com) so your loved one can receive emails and photos from the family without having to use a computer. This is an especially wonderful tool for people who would enjoy a snapshot of their grandchild at the park earlier that afternoon or to receive a photo from an adult child who is visiting a place that the older adult had visited with them in the past.

- Accompany your loved one to a movie, visit a public garden, go to the library to check out a classical music CD, or organize any other outing that has been customary and can be sustained. If your loved one has typically gone to the corner store to have a cup of coffee and read the newspaper, you can be instrumental in sustaining this ritual. This can bring connectedness, predictability and a sense of accomplishment.

- In order to promote stimulation of the mind, creativity or idea exchange, simply engage the person in conversation about their work history, their first car, their favorite subjects in school, favorite foods, or other topics that might be explored when getting to know someone. Reminiscence activity cards are available as are mental fitness cards that are full of ideas about 'brain aerobics.'

- Even for those who have no history of creative expression through art, it may be surprising to see how a set of colored pencils or watercolors and an invitation to see how the colors look on the paper sets off the imagination or provides an opportunity for expression when words and/or memories may be more elusive. The Alzheimer Association's Memories in the Making program has enjoyed great success in engaging clients with memory changes in creating art by using an "inspiration piece" and encouraging the client to copy an appealing image.

- Many communities offer an abundance of lectures, performances and senior center programming that can be easily discovered by regularly perusing the local newspaper. Take responsibility for reviewing the newspaper with your loved one to discuss options and create a plan to attend an event of interest. For many seniors, physical or cognitive limitations may make it difficult to rely on outings, community events or other people for opportunities to engage. For all, there is an opportunity to try to make 'down time' at home more engaging.

- Create a customized therapeutic activity kit. This type of box (or basket, bin, etc.) contains activities that can be implemented by family members to stimulate the mind. Examples of items that might go in a therapeutic activity kit include letters in plastic coverings that can be read and reread regularly, music CDs, art supplies, postcards from places where the client has traveled, playing cards, balls or fabrics with different textures to help stimulate touch and photos or other items that trigger pleasant memories and cognitive response. The most important aspect of creating a therapeutic activity kit is considering the individual needs, interests and capabilities of the person for whom the kit is created. Therapeutic activity kits can be created by a family member or a professional, such as a geriatric care manager or recreational therapist.

- Cultivating spirituality can be done by helping someone connect to anything that gives them a sense of purpose and meaning. For some, the ritual of churchgoing provides an outlet to create order and build faith despite frustrating and sometimes painful health challenges that cause them to need care. For others, a connection with nature by sitting by the ocean and watching the waves, hearing the water and feeling the breeze, or working in the garden to continue cultivating the roses out front that are celebrated by homeowner and neighbors alike can be equally as powerful.

Activities for Seniors with Dementia

Dementia robs a person of his cognitive function, often leaving behind what seems to be nothing but a shell of the one who you knew and loved. Many people with late stage dementia spend most of their days sleeping or staring off into space. Often it is possible to engage the person in other activities. If you are caring for a loved one with dementia, this section provides a few tips for initiating activities.

- Keep to a general schedule. Most people with dementia like to know what they can expect out of each day. They may become anxious or angry if their routine varies too much.

- Schedule times for personal hygiene, meals, exercise and other active pursuits, as well as time for naps.

- Encourage the person with dementia to do as much as possible for himself, even if an activity takes longer that way.

- Don't give the person a chance to refuse. Use positive language and encouragement. For instance, do not say, "Would you like to eat?" Instead say, "It's time for lunch."

- Keep instructions simple and short, and give each instruction one at a time.

- Offer choices between no more than two selections. If you offer a wider range of choices, the person may become confused and upset. ("Would you like to wear your blue shirt or your red shirt today?")

- Don't be afraid to make activities a little challenging. If your loved one shows signs of becoming agitated, stop that activity and shift his attention to something else.

- Avoid activities and conversations that rely on short-term memory. Most people with dementia have much clearer memories of the distant past.

- Limit stimulation. One or two visitors are fine, but a roomful is too many. Likewise, don't try to play dominoes with your loved one while the television is blaring, the dog is barking to go out, and the oven timer is going off.

- Keep a few favorite items or activities stowed away to use if your loved one starts getting upset. Agree with whatever your loved one is saying, and redirect his attention to the favorite item.

- Never argue or get into verbal disagreements.

Carefully selected activities can help keep seniors stay psychologically engaged and at peace with their lives. The next chapter focuses on the psychology of the home bound patient, including certain disordered behaviors that may appear, and how you should consider handling these types of situations.

FIVE

Psychology of Home Bound Seniors

While in nursing school, Daphne Neilson was instructed to go home and put on an adult diaper. She was told to wear that diaper for the next 10 hours without a break, to mimic the experience had by those seniors who do not have the personal attention of a caregiver to change them frequently. It was an unusual experience.

The entire class came in the next morning notably affected. The experiment brought out different feelings in everyone: fear, discomfort, humiliation, anger, and ultimately understanding. Not a single nursing student ever viewed those adult diapers the same way. The experiment remains a constant reminder of how deeply personal and important the role that caregiving is for those under care.

People who need live-in care may experience a wide variety of emotions, depending on their circumstances and their temperament before they became ill or injured. One way to understand some of the feelings that a person with a debilitating illness or injury might experience is to look at Elisabeth Kubler-Ross' five stages of grief.

Elisabeth Kubler-Ross: Five Stages of Grief

Years ago, Kubler-Ross broke the medical taboo of mentioning death to dying patients. She not only told her patients when they were dying but also encouraged them to talk about their feelings.

Her resulting observations, which have become known as the five stages of grief, have been popular in the social sciences for many years. Though the five stages have recently been questioned in bereavement literature, they remain pertinent when applied to patients.

When studying the five stages, it is important to remember that each individual has a different experience of grieving the loss of his or her own health. Many will go through some or all of the emotions that Kubler-Ross identifies, but not necessarily in the prescribed order. Some will remain stuck in one stage, while others will veer back and forth among the stages. Some people may even identify different feelings entirely.

Although the five stages of grief may help you understand how a loved one reacts to their life changes, do not try to impose this model on your family as the only method of healthy grieving. People who suddenly become paralyzed, learn that they have a terminal disease or suffer major acute illnesses suffer incredible shock at how their life circumstances have changed. Kubler-Ross is a generalized grief reaction model; it is not a "perfect" model.

Denial

The first stage identified by Kubler-Ross is denial. People who have suffered a sudden decline in health may deny the reality of their condition. "I just don't feel like going out today. I'll do the shopping next week." Or, "What do those stupid doctors know? I tell you, I'm going to walk again."

The best way to handle denial is to listen supportively without reinforcing the wishful thinking. For instance, if the person you are caring for has a terminal illness, and says "I'll be taking that cruise to Greece next summer," an appropriate response might be, "I know how you've always wanted to go there. How did you get so interested in it?" or "That would be just wonderful, wouldn't it?"

Avoid confronting the person with their denial ("You'll never make it on another trip") and avoid playing into the fantasy ("Of course you'll go to Greece next summer. Let's book those tickets now.").

Anger

The second stage of grief is anger. There are many possible targets for anger. The person may be angry at the illness or injury, at God, at the doctors who failed to restore health, or at everything else. Unfortunately, your loved one may even take out their anger on you.

In general, most people are grateful for the care they receive, although some people tend to resent needing it and, by extension, to resent the caregiver who is providing it. Many experience anger and frustration at not being able to do the things they used to do.

The most important thing you can do is to hold your temper in the face of anger. If you do feel yourself becoming angry and about to become engaged in a confrontation, take a few deep breaths, count to ten, or step out of the room until you are sure you can approach your loved one in a calm, respectful manner. Try to respond to anger with empathy and support. For example, use comments such as, "I know this has got to be really hard for you. Is there anything I can do to make it easier?"

It is also important to realize, however, that you do not deserve to be emotionally or physically abused by anyone. If a loved one becomes abusive, identify the behavior and say it isn't acceptable. If you can safely do so, leave them alone for a little while to calm down. For instance, you might say, "I know you're angry now, but I won't let you call me names. I'll be back to check on you in a little while."

Bargaining

Kubler-Ross noticed that many of her dying patients go through a stage of grief during which they appear to be trying to strike a bargain with God, or the universe: "I'll be super-nice to everyone and maybe God will make me well again." Or, "I'll do penance for past mistakes, I'll stop drinking, I'll forgive my sister who stole from me, I'll become a doctor and save other lives…"

Sometimes bargaining takes the form of asking for just a little more time. "I don't mind dying as long as I get to see my granddaughter graduate from high school first." Many individuals attempt to bargain with their doctors. "Maybe just one more round of chemotherapy would turn things around" or "I think if I stayed another week in rehab I could probably go home by myself."

Most of the time these statements require nothing more than empathetic listening. You don't want to rob your loved one of hope, but neither do you want to instill false hope, so let them talk and then make non-committal responses like, "I hear you," or "I know how much you want to get better." You don't need to tell your loved one that the bargains won't work—they'll figure that out independently.

If the bargaining involves the medical team, let your loved one's doctor be the one to explain why additional chemotherapy would be more harmful than helpful or why another week in rehabilitation would have no added benefit.

One type of bargaining that can be especially difficult for caregivers to listen to is self-recrimination. Rather than making deals for the future, some bargainers carefully examine the past in an attempt to affix blame. Sometimes the blame lands on another party who caused their injury. All too often, though, the bargainer reaches the conclusion that they are defective and somehow to blame. If the bargaining takes this form, you might hear statements like, "God must be punishing me for something," or "It's my own fault. I was the one who wouldn't stop smoking."

It's human nature to want to rush in with reassurances: "Of course God isn't punishing you, that's not how he works," or "You tried to quit smoking a thousand times. You did the best you could." While both of these statements may be true, they also ignore the pain being felt. Instead of disputing the facts, acknowledge the emotions. "It's got to be painful to feel as if this is somehow your fault." Again, most people reach their own peace with the blame issue without much help or prompting from you.

Depression/Sadness

Kubler-Ross calls her fourth stage in the grief process depression. For purposes of this book, we are going to call it "sadness" in order to differentiate it from clinical depression, which requires psychological intervention and treatment.

At some point in this process, your loved one will realize that they are now home bound and that the situation probably won't change significantly over time. There will be no trip to Greece in the summer, no new physical therapist who will come charging in on a white horse and restore full mobility – in other words, no miraculous cure.

The natural result of such a significant life change is sadness. You may notice that your loved one has become very quiet. You may see tears or a change in appetite or sleeping patterns. Your loved one may also stop performing enjoyable activities or the activities of daily living still within his or her grasp.

Your approach to sadness should be threefold. First, develop an attitude of watching and waiting. If the sadness persists beyond a couple of weeks, or appears to be growing worse, chances are you are dealing with clinical depression.

Second, offer your loved one comfort and support. This does not mean that you should try to "cheer your loved one up." Instead, offer quiet presence and empathetic listening. If words are necessary, you might say something like, "I can't even begin to understand how you must feel, but I want you to know we will get through this. Together."

Third, insist that your loved one continue to participate in activities of daily living as long as he or she is still capable. You may feel like a bully at first, but it's perfectly possible to be both gentle and firm. "Mom, push up with your legs when I lift you. Otherwise, we might both fall and get hurt." Or, "Dad, I need you to shave yourself. You know I always cut you when I try to shave you, so please help me out."

Acceptance

Some people reach the point emotionally at which they are able to accept their change to home bound status without significant emotional trauma. A man with heart disease, for instance, said, "What's to miss about going outside? It's too cold in the winter and too hot in the summer, and now that my kids all grown, I've finally talked my sons into mowing the lawn."

Your heart is guaranteed to leap the first time you hear your loved one make neutral or even positive statements about being home bound. A word of caution: People often cycle through the various stages of grief many times. Just because Mom appears to have reached acceptance today doesn't mean she won't be angry tomorrow or sad for two weeks after that. Just as our own moods are rarely static, your loved one's feelings about their situation will change day-to-day and over time.

Five Stages of Grief with Multiple Sclerosis

Mabelene Pepito, RN, BSN, of Home Care Assistance in Danville, California, shares the story of Sarah, a 69-year-old woman who had been dealing with Multiple Sclerosis for over 15 years. The MS has confined her to a wheel chair and she could no longer care for herself. Getting dressed, going to the bathroom, and eating was difficult for her. Her family could no longer be there for her 24 hours a day so they hired a caregiver to help. Here is Mabelene's account of Sarah's journey through the 5 stages of grief:

Denial:

"When I first came in, Sarah was going through some physical therapy to help get some control back in her hands and legs. She would tell me that with all this therapy, she will be able to walk that marathon as she did in her past. All I could do to help her was to listen and be a supportive voice in continuing her therapy. I did not have to say much to her but tell her that it would be nice to get her to walk that marathon as she did in her past."

Anger:
"Even after all the physical therapy she was doing, she could not regain control again of her extremities. Her frustration showed the most during meal times and she would drop her food on her clothes or not being able to get the food into her mouth. She would curse and say mean things to me and other caregivers who were trying to help her. She would even get so angry that she would throw the plate on to the floor. When she became that way, I would clean up what I can off her clothes and attempt to calm her down and let her talk through the anger. After expressing her anger, she would request to be alone and calm herself down. Only then she would attempt to eat a simple meal again."

Bargaining:
"Sarah would often say that she wished she knew how this happened to her. She would go back and say if she lived a healthier life style, she would not be in this condition. She would even say that if she was a better mother, she would be able to do more things for herself and not rely on her children so much. During that time, all I could do was give an attentive ear and let her know that her feelings were understood."

Depression:
"There were weeks when I came in to Sarah's room and she refused to get out of bed. She covered her face with her blanket and did not want any help. She would only pick at her meals and

needed to be encouraged to drink fluids. At times, I would even hear her crying from under her blanket. During those times, all I could do was be there for her. I would make sure she ate and drank her fluids. After a day or two, I would then try to sit with her and let her talk. Little words and simple hand holding made her come out from under the blanket. Once she came out from under the blanket, I would encourage more conversation. And again provide an attentive ear. Once I helped her to sit up in the bed, I would then attempt to get her dressed. It took time to get her to do those things but once she recovered, she would have a smile on her face."

Acceptance:
"When Sarah had her good days, she would be joyful, smiling and even laughing. She would love to get out and sit in the lobby during the summer weather. She also loved to tell stories of her life and kids. She was a great storyteller and even told some stories that she felt were funny when she was diagnosed with the MS. She would say, 'I could get used to having someone take care of me. I am now the queen and I have you at my fingertips."

"Sarah's health continued to decline. She could not get out of bed anymore and we would go through more of the depressed days. It was important that Sarah had her routine and her set place in her bed. Flowers at her bedside, a glass of water with a straw, her favorite book at the end of her pillow and the picture of her children and grandchildren in her view. Every day at the end of my shift, she would hold my hand, give it a kiss and tell me how much she loved our time together. I always made sure there was a smile on my face."

Clinical Depression

It is important that you know how to distinguish between clinical depression and the more commonly experienced reactive depression that is a response to being shut in at home or even bed bound. Reactive depression feels bad, but clinical depression can be life threatening.

Clinical depression is more than just a case of "the blues." It goes beyond the understandable sadness one feels when trying to cope with the burden of declining health. Clinical depression, sometimes called major depression, is a pattern of mood and behavioral symptoms that last at least two weeks and often much longer.

According to the Mayo Clinic, symptoms of clinical depression extend beyond merely having a sad or downcast mood. People who are seriously depressed are often irritable and so lost in their own pain that they have little patience with others. Additionally, people with major depression tend to lose interest in activities they used to enjoy.

Depression also wreaks havoc on the sleep cycle and the appetite. Some people who are depressed want to sleep all the time. For many, sleep becomes a means of escape from the harsh realities of life. Others with depression, however, will develop insomnia and will toss and turn for hours worrying about their condition. Eating habits can also be affected by clinical depression. Some people who are depressed can't seem to stop eating and others can't be persuaded to take a bite.

If your loved one is clinically depressed, you may also notice cognitive impairment. In fact, cognitive impairments can be so pronounced that the person may be misdiagnosed with dementia instead of depression. In general, people who are depressed think, talk, and move very slowly, as if every word is an effort. They may also have trouble making decisions, and they may be easily distractible and unable to handle complex tasks.

Some people who are depressed develop what is called "agitated depression." Instead of moving and talking slowly, they can't seem to sit still. The older adult with agitated depression may spend a lot of time pacing or wandering through the home. If your loved one is confined to a bed or a wheelchair, you might notice symptoms like the wringing of hands, playing with bedcovers or clothing, or a constant tapping of the feet. A person with agitated depression may also experience "flight of thought," meaning they cannot follow the normal flow of conversation and instead jump from topic to topic in ways that often make no sense to others.

Another common symptom of clinical depression is feeling guilty or worthless. For many seniors, these feelings may be reinforced by circumstances. "I'm nothing but trouble to my daughter—see how hard she has to work to take care of me." Or, "My husband had to take early retirement to take care of me. I'm ruining his life."

Perhaps the most difficult form of clinical depression is the one that is most common. Oddly, many people in society accept this kind of thinking as sound and reasonable. The thing to remember, however, is that the wish to die is never normal and always associated with depression – no matter how it is couched.

Clinical depression negatively impacts the person suffering from it as well as the people who care for them. If you suspect your loved one suffers from major depression, seek professional help as soon as possible.

Depression Interventions

If you notice signs of depression in your loved one, talk with them about their feelings. Older adults have often grown up with a significant stigma surrounding mental health disorders. They don't like to think of themselves as depressed. An older adult will probably respond best to questions like, "You seem kind of blue lately, what's going on?" or "Is it hard for you to focus on your books? I noticed you haven't been reading as much as usual."

Your next step is to talk to your doctor. He may prescribe an antidepressant medication to alleviate symptoms. For many people, antidepressants can bring about improvements in energy levels and mood in two to four weeks. They are not, however, magic bullets. It takes medication awhile to become fully effective. Furthermore, the first antidepressant a doctor tries might not work. Finding the right medication is often a matter of trial and error.

If your loved one is receiving home care services, ask if a care manager can make regular visits to assess for depression symptoms. You may also want to contact your local senior center or your local Area Agency on Aging to see if they know of any mental health professionals that will work with older adults.

If religion plays an important part in your loved one's life, the priest, minister, rabbi, or imam from your place of worship can be persuaded to visit and provide a little extra emotional support.

Dos and Don'ts for Talking to Someone Who is Depressed

DO treat your loved one with the same respect that you always have. You needn't talk baby talk or shield them from unpleasant truths.

DO acknowledge the depression and praise any efforts your loved one makes. "I can tell just getting up is a real effort. I'm so proud of you for doing it."

DO try to keep some sort of regular schedule. Ask your loved one to help you around the house in some small way. Discourage sleeping too much during the daytime, as this can lead to insomnia at night.

DO encourage your loved one to take part in activities and make choices. Getting started is the hardest part for people who are depressed. Once they're engaged, they'll usually stick with an activity for a little while.

DO tell the person how much he or she is loved.

DO reach out to your loved one. If he or she rebuffs you at first, reach out again and again.

DO offer to listen if your loved one wants to talk. Listen quietly and respectfully without providing advice or attempting to trivialize his or her feelings.

DON'T tell your loved one to "Get over it!" or "Snap out of it." No one wants to be depressed. If your loved one could snap out of it, they would.

DON'T tell your loved one that other people are much worse off. Comparing pain isn't useful.

DON'T imply that your loved one is lazy, selfish, or weak. Instead, take note of the positive things your loved one says or does, and encourage those behaviors with praise.

DON'T tell your loved one to "turn it over to God" or that if their faith was stronger, they wouldn't be depressed. People of all religious faiths experience depression.

Anxiety and Seniors

People who require live-in care usually experience a great deal of anxiety. Some are afraid of specific things: "What if a burglar breaks into the home while my daughter is at work?" "What if my caregiver doesn't get me to the bathroom in time and I have an accident in bed?" "What if the electricity goes off and my oxygen stops working?"

Other seniors experience what is called free-floating anxiety. They're upset and worried, but they can't tell you exactly what they're worried about. Or perhaps they focus on one concern, but as soon as that concern is addressed, they turn their fears to something else.

Individuals with problems that affect their breathing tend to be especially prone to anxiety, especially if their disease makes them feel as if they cannot catch their breath.

Micah Garibay, Senior Staffing Coordinator of Home Care Assistance in Palo Alto, California, remembers taking care of a woman with respiratory problems. When nighttime fell and her caregivers left for the day, the women would call the agency for reassurance. Sometimes she would call the agency five or six times a night. Her complaints were always different. Sometimes she thought her little dog was sick. Once she complained her oxygen wasn't working, but it actually was. A few times she was afraid she would run out of her medicine. "She was so scared to be alone," Micah remembers. "We eventually had her caregivers stay with her through the night so she wouldn't worry."

The best way to deal with anxiety that is spiraling out of control is to address the root cause of the problem. Pick a time when you and the person you are caring for are getting along well. Sit close and say something like, "I can't imagine how hard it must be for you to have to be here all by yourself. I know you get really scared. Let's see if we can figure out a way to help you feel more secure."

Then let the person talk. Your loved one probably has many ideas about what would help them feel less fearful. Here are a few additional suggestions:

- **Establish a ritual to follow whenever you leave the person alone.** This might include helping him to the bathroom, making sure he has water and food available, putting a book or the television remote control within his reach, and telling him exactly where you are going and when you will be back.

- **Make sure your loved one can contact someone if an emergency occurs.** You might place a telephone or a cell phone within reach, or help him obtain a personal medical alarm so they can summon help with the push of a button.

- **Re-arrange the environment.** This may mean installing a home security system so your loved one will feel safer while you are gone. Or it may involve moving living quarters to the main floor so he or she has easier access to other rooms in the house. You might also consider asking your doctor about durable medical equipment. A hospital bed, for instance, gives people a lot more control than a regular bed. Consider a urinal and a bedside commode to make getting to the bathroom easier.

- **Keep the person occupied.** Seniors often manufacture anxiety when they are bored. After being alone for hours, every sound becomes exaggerated and every vague threat becomes immediate and deadly. For example, the person who kept calling a neighbor in the middle of the night, can't sleep. She would lie in the dark thinking of all the terrible things that might happen to her. Her friend arranged for her to get a television in her bedroom and helped her purchase some craft projects she could work on when sleep wouldn't come. Once her friend made this arrangement, the number of calls dropped dramatically.

- **Introduce relaxation techniques.** When your loved one begins to get agitated, force yourself to remain calm. Ask him to take five slow, deep breaths with you. Encourage him to focus on relaxing his body. Lower and deepen your voice to encourage him to do the same. When he is calmer, help him figure out what caused the anxiety and try to avoid that trigger in the future.

- **Ask about medication.** Because anti-anxiety medications and sleeping medications tend to be habit-forming and interact with other drugs, doctors are hesitant to prescribe them for seniors.

Many doctors, however, will make an exception for older adults with a chronic or terminal illness. If your loved one is prescribed medication, make sure he takes it at the first sign of anxiety and not in the midst of a full-blown panic attack. If you have concerns, always discuss them with your loved one's physician.

Conclusion

If you suspect possible mental illness, two organizations that provide excellent support for family members are the National Alliance on Mental Illness (NAMI) in the United States and the Canadian Mental Health Association in Canada. Both organizations have chapters and support groups in most major cities. You can learn more through their websites, http://nami.org and http://cmha.ca

Now that you're aware of some of the psychological characteristics of older adults, the next chapter looks at several common issues faced by people who are confined to the home by illness or injury.

SIX

Challenges and Special Circumstances

No two home bound seniors are exactly alike. Each person presents a unique set of challenges and issues. However, there are a few problem areas that are common. This chapter looks at these obstacles and offers positive ways to resolve these issues.

Lack of Mobility/Deconditioning

Most home bound seniors have some level of mobility. Some get around by doing what is called the "furniture walk," or holding onto furniture for support as they move around their homes. Others use a walker, a cane, or sometimes a pair of crutches. Some home bound seniors are less mobile, and use either a wheelchair or a scooter to get around.

Some of these less mobile seniors can move themselves (transfer) from the wheelchair to the toilet or the bed. Others need the help of one or more caregivers to assist them. Finally, a significant number of people confined to the home are also confined to the bed and require a mechanical lift for transfers

Seniors who are unable to move their arms and legs easily are likely to experience wasting and weakness of the muscles. This is called "deconditioning." Deconditioning is sometimes the natural result of a disease process, such as muscular dystrophy, and will occur no matter what the caregiver does. Other times, deconditioning can be slowed or prevented by assisting the individual with simple exercises.

Bedsores (Decubitus Ulcers, Pressure Ulcers)

Bed or pressure sores are serious problems for seniors who are bed bound. They grow quickly and can even lead to death if not treated promptly. Bed sores occur when a person with limited mobility experiences damage to the skin and the underlying tissue due to pressure. Pressure sores usually occur in places on the body where the weight rests against a mattress or other surface, such as the seat of a chair or wheelchair. Pressure sores are common on the bottom and on the heels.

Some people, especially those who are severely deconditioned and malnourished—will get bedsores no matter what the caregiver does. However, there are several steps that a caregiver can take to reduce the likelihood of bedsores.

Checking the skin

Whenever you help, bathe or dress your loved one, carefully check the skin for red areas and places where the skin appears scabbed or there are open wounds. Report any of these abnormalities to your doctor.

Repositioning

Repositioning means helping a bed or chair bound person shift positions every one to two hours. This is accomplished by moving the person from the left to the right side. Pillows can be used for support and to help hold the position. If the senior is in a wheelchair, you can reposition them slightly by having them shift their weight from one buttock to the other, again using pillows for support. Because sitting places more pressure on the tailbone than lying down, the person in a wheelchair should spend at least part of the day in bed.

Keep the skin clean

If your loved one is incontinent, be sure to wash and dry the genital area, the area between the thighs, and their bottom after each episode of incontinence. There are some products that act as a barrier between the skin and moisture and you should consider using one of these. Seniors with urinary incontinence can sometimes avoid bedsores by using an indwelling catheter. Again, this is a decision you should make with your doctor.

"Float" the heels

If the skin on the heels is breaking down, encourage your loved one to lie on their side. If they are unable or unwilling to do so, place a couple of pillows under their calves to elevate their feet off the mattress.

Change mattresses

Some mattresses, such as low air loss mattresses or egg crate mattresses, reduce the risk of bedsores. These mattresses are provided by medical supply stores and usually require a doctor's order. Medicare will cover the cost of a special mattress in many cases. Some private insurance companies also will pay for these special mattresses.

Maintain good nutrition

By adding protein to the diet with special shakes like Ensure or Boost, you can help avoid bedsores. Caregivers should also encourage foods high in protein, like lean meats, fish, peanut butter, cheese, most types of beans, and eggs. Any of these diet changes will help seniors avoid bedsores.

Falls

Falls happen in many ways. A senior who is able to walk, although unsteadily, might slip on a slick floor or trip over a small object or simply lose their balance. If your loved one has severe osteoporosis, their hip might break simply from the weight of the body (this is called a pathological fracture), leading to a tumble. A senior who is confined to a wheelchair or to bed might fall when leaning over to reach for something on the floor or on a nearby table. Some seniors with dementia become confused and try to stand up on their own, believing they can walk.

Most falls can happen in the blink of an eye. Although they can and do occur while the caregiver is out of the house or in another room, many occur right in front of the caregiver, who feels powerless to stop them. Even though falls are not 100% preventable, there are some things you can do to decrease their likelihood. There are also some steps you can take to minimize the damage if a fall does occur.

Keep walkways clear

If you have children in the house, make sure they don't leave toys or objects on the floor. Other items that can cause falls include clothes or towels on the floor, accent rugs, and electrical power cords stretched across a hallway or doorway. Always wipe up spills immediately to avoid slips on a wet surface.

Remind your loved one to use assistive devices

If the doctor recommends that your loved one get around with a walker or cane, make sure they use it.

Install handrails to reduce the risk of falls while toileting or bathing
Handrails are available at most pharmacies, medical equipment and discount stores. They are easy to install or can be installed through a local contractor or medical supply store.

Check clothing and shoes
Avoid such clothing as long bathrobes that drag on the ground and get caught under feet. Shoes and slippers should fit comfortably and have non-skid soles. Discourage walking around barefoot.

Keep things close at hand
Keep items your loved one uses frequently, like a glass of water, the television remote control, a bell to summon you, and a box of tissues right beside the bed or chair within easy reach.

Consider getting a tray table for the wheelchair
This will prevent your loved one from standing up or leaning out of the chair. Because it is a type of restraint, however, you'll want to discuss the pros and cons of using one with your doctor.

Talk to your doctor about bedrails
Like a tray table, bedrails are considered a form of restraint. If your loved one is determined to climb out of bed, bedrails can actually cause injury if they get tangled or fall. Other options include concave mattresses, which have sides that curve upward to prevent rolling out of bed, and bolster overlays, which provide soft barriers to discourage the your loved one from getting up on their own.

Purchase a bed or chair alarm

There are two kinds of alarms. One senses pressure and alerts if the pressure is removed (i.e., if your loved one gets up). The other is a two part alarm. One part is safety-pinned to clothing and the other part is attached to the chair or bed. The two parts are then connected by a magnet. If your loved one stands up, he breaks the magnetic connection and a loud alarm sounds.

As mentioned above, in spite of your best efforts, your loved one may still fall. There are a few things you can do to lessen the risk of injury.

Lower your loved one to the ground

If you observe a fall, don't try to stop it from happening. If you do, you're likely to get injured, too. Instead, grab your loved one under the arms or by the gait belt and gently lower them to the floor. Don't hesitate to call 911 for assistance.

Remove furniture with sharp corners

Many falls happen at night, when trying to get out of bed to go to the bathroom. If there is a table with sharp corners beside the bed, your loved one may hit his head on it on the way down, causing a head injury as well as other bumps and bruises from the fall. An alternative to removing the furniture entirely is to tie towels around the corners to cushion them.

Get a personal medical alarm

Popularized by the commercial where a woman cries, "I've fallen and I can't get up," these alarms work through your phone system. Your loved one wears a waterproof bracelet or necklace with an alarm button. In the event of a fall or other injury, a simple push of a button summons 911, family, friends, or neighbors. This is especially important if your loved one lives alone. Remaining on the floor for hours can cause just as much damage as the fall itself.

Discourage moving after a fall

If your loved one falls, encourage them to lie still while you check for obvious injuries such as bleeding head wounds and limbs that are bent in the wrong direction. If everything looks all right, gently move his arms and legs and ask him to tell you if anything hurts. Then have him get to his hands and knees and try to lift himself off the floor while you use a gait belt to assist.

Call 911

If your loved one is injured or in pain or cannot get off the floor easily, call 911. At the very least, the paramedics will help you get your loved one back into bed or a wheelchair. They may also recommend going to the emergency room for x-rays and observation.

Notify the doctor, home care agency, or hospice after every fall. Even if your loved one does not appear to be injured, his healthcare team may want to take a second look to be sure.

Burns

Burns can occur when a confused individual attempts to use appliances in the kitchen. Debra Stanson, a hospice social worker, remembers one client who tried to microwave her adult diapers in order to dry them. A fire started in the microwave, and when the woman tried to open the door to put it out, she burned her hands.

If your loved one has been diagnosed with Alzheimer's disease or another form of dementia, do not leave them in the kitchen alone. Supervise any use of the stove or oven, just as you would do with a child who doesn't know how to cook safely. If you and your loved one cook meals together, make sure you are the last one to leave the kitchen. Don't go until you are sure all the appliances are turned off.

Some people with Alzheimer's continue to live alone or stay alone for a time. All too often, caregivers report arriving home to find the gas stove on or food burned to a crisp in the oven or toaster. You can help avoid incidents like this by disabling the stove and oven and unplugging other appliances like the toaster and the microwave. Then make sure to leave meals that your loved one can enjoy without heating them up, like a peanut butter sandwich or a fruit salad. You may also want to arrange for Meals on Wheels or a similar group to deliver nutritious food.

Pain and Physical Symptoms

Seniors may experience pain or discomfort from many sources. People who have been injured in an accident may continue to experience pain from their injuries for a long time. Illnesses like cancer or HIV are often responsible for pain. People with lung and heart diseases may not have a lot of pain, but they may have trouble catching their breath, which is just as unpleasant. In addition, some people suffer from pain that has nothing to do with their primary diagnosis. Many seniors, for instance, suffer from old injuries, chronic arthritis, and neuropathy (nerve damage that causes a tingling sensation) in the extremities.

You should feel free to ask about pain yourself. Ask your loved one, "Do you hurt anywhere?" If the answer is yes, ask where the pain is and have them describe it (sharp, dull, pinching, burning, etc.) and rate it on a scale of one to ten, with one being almost no pain and ten being the worst pain.

Because your loved one might be reluctant to admit to being in pain, also watch for nonverbal signs and symptoms: facial grimacing, moaning, restlessness, limping, gasping with sudden movement, crying out, etc. Keep your doctor informed about any pain your loved one reports or exhibits and ask what you can do to make the symptoms better. There are many kinds of medications, some narcotic and some not, that can be used to treat pain. Some doctors also prescribe home remedies, like gentle massage for stiff muscles, a hot pack to an aching neck or ice to dull the pain of a sprained wrist. Follow your doctor's treatment instructions and report back with the results.

If your loved one continues to exhibit pain or discomfort, has a life-limiting condition like cancer or end-stage Alzheimer's, and has stopped curative treatment for the illness, consider a referral to hospice for symptom management. A senior who does not have a terminal condition may be referred to a pain management clinic if their primary care doctor can't get the pain under control.

Abuse, Neglect, and Exploitation

Abuse is a behavior directed against another person that is intended to cause harm. Abuse can be physical, like slapping, kicking, whipping, or burning. It can also be emotional, such as name-calling, making threats, or telling lies to frighten someone. In addition abuse can be sexual, such as fondling the genitals of a person who does not or cannot give consent; rape; and making inappropriate sexual remarks. Neglect means failing to provide care that a person needs to survive and thrive. It can involve a failure to provide food, recommended medical care, and assistance with personal hygiene. In addition, exploitation means misusing another person's resources to benefit oneself, such as stealing a family member's social security check or convincing a demented person to write out a large check from their bank account.

According to the National Center on Elder Abuse, between one and two million American seniors are mistreated or exploited by a caregiver each year. Of these cases, only about one in 14 come to the attention of police or social service agencies.

Home bound individuals are uniquely vulnerable to abuse, neglect, and exploitation for several reasons. First, because they are not mobile, they may have little contact with the outside world and no ability to tell a sympathetic person that they are being mistreated. Second, home bound seniors are likely to have psychological conditions such as depression, anger, and anxiety. An inexperienced caregiver may respond with anger or negligence. Third, many home bound seniors require extensive care that their caregiver doesn't know how to provide or is physically unable to provide. In addition, home bound seniors often live with family members who are barely getting by financially. The family may need the loved one's social security check to make their house payment.

The next chapter will discuss stress and steps a live-in caregiver can take to make life a little easier.

SEVEN

Tips for the Live-in Caregiver

Many people who are currently providing live-in care for a parent or relative did not expect to become caregivers. Some would probably even have denied it was possible that it could happen to them.

As one daughter described it, "One minute you're minding your own business, living a life you enjoy. The next minute, the phone rings and it's the hospital, or you get an email from your Mom's neighbor saying that your Mom is doing the gardening in her nightgown. And just like that, you disappear, and your life as a caregiver begins." When an unexpected event like the one just described turns your life upside down, it's normal to have feelings of ambivalence, anger, and frustration. You may resent the person who needs care, even if it's not their fault.

Ambivalence

When it first becomes clear that your loved one is going to need ongoing care and that you will be the person primarily responsible for providing it, your first feeling will might be ambivalence. On the one hand, you might think, 'I'll do anything I can for Mom. After all, she took care of me.' On the other hand, you might think, "But how will I make time to give Mom all the help she needs?" Ambivalence can lead to feelings of shame: "What kind of daughter am I, anyway. How can I be so ungrateful?"

Ambivalence, however, is perfectly normal when facing any kind of life change, especially one that is not of your choosing. The best way to handle ambivalence is to acknowledge it and be willing to gather with other family members, ask the hard questions, and solicit their assistance and advice. You might find that you don't have to take on all the responsibility for caregiving.

Resentment and Anger

Your life has been turned upside down and you have a lot to be angry about. You might be angry with your loved one for being frail or ill. You might be angry with other family members that don't step up and help. You might even be angry at God or at the doctors who weren't able to help your loved one.

Once again, these feelings are normal. Find a trusted friend, member of the clergy, mental health professional, support group, or family member and talk about the anger and resentment you are feeling. If you resent your loved one, it's probably better not to express those feelings to them. Once you fall into a caregiving routine and find the support you need, your resentment usually lessens, though it may never go away altogether.

A word of warning: if you are angry at your loved one and resent them to the point where you have thoughts of hurting them, physically or emotionally, you need to step out of the role of caregiver. In situations like this, home care agencies can make a world of difference to your mental health.

Embarrassment

One family caregiver said, "Now it's old hat, but the first time I had to give my mother a bath, I went to my room and cried for an hour." Being a caregiver often means providing your loved one with the most intimate care imaginable: bathing, examining skin for pressure ulcers, cleaning the genital area, changing diapers, and more.

No matter what the relationship is between you and the person needing care, these moments can be awkward and embarrassing. If either party is truly humiliated by having a loved one provide personal care, the family might want to consider hiring a caregiver from a home care agency like Home Care Assistance to handle the more intimate aspects of caregiving.

Frustration

At one time or another, your loved one is likely to develop one or more behaviors that you will find extremely frustrating. Maybe you're an upbeat person by nature and your loved one has sunk into a deep depression. Maybe your loved one gets into your private papers, or gossips with her friends about your love life, or refuses to follow the diet the doctor ordered.

When you're feeling frustrated, the most therapeutic and beneficial step you can take is to seek out another caregiver or caregiver support group. Find an individual, or multiple individuals, who understands what you are going through and who can offer valuable advice.

Inflexibility

Caregivers often develop strict routines that help get them through the day. For example, the caregiver serves their client breakfast at exactly 9:00 A.M. each day. Laundry is always finished and put away by 10:30 A.M. The senior then helps out with small household chores until it is time for lunch.

There is no problem with developing a routine. People who require caregiving generally like knowing what is going to happen and when. It takes some of the uncertainty and fear out of their day and gives them a sense of control.

Problems can occur, however, if you stick so closely to your schedule that a single interruption or change of plan spoils the entire day. Being inflexible about routines can also make it harder for others to help you, because they are unlikely to do things exactly as you would.

Debra Stanson, who works with hospice patients, recalled a caregiver who was becoming overwhelmed with the amount of care her father needed. Debra located a volunteer respite program in the area that would provide caregivers four hours per day, two times per week, so that the daughter could take a break. The next time Debra visited the family, she asked the daughter how the respite care was going.

"Oh, I put a stop to that," the daughter said. "That girl wouldn't do what I told her!" "In what way?" Debra asked. "She put the towels on the left side of the cabinet instead of the right side." Debra was unable to convince the caregiver that this small slip from routine, which could be remedied in a moment's time, was not a good reason to reject the whole service.

If you see yourself in this story, take a step back and let others help you. True, they may feed your parent at 9:30 A.M. instead of 9:00 A.M. and yes, you might find blue socks in the drawer instead of white socks but, overall, these are insignificant details. This shouldn't prevent you from getting help from others who mean well and want to make your life easier.

Loss of Self

Being the caregiver of an older adult can be a full-time job. If you let it, it can consume your whole life. You have no other role except "the caregiver." You forget that you are also a wife, mom, CPA, or a member of your local church.

Yes, being a caregiver is a significant part of your identity now, but you are much more than just that. Be sure to take time each day, even if it's just a few minutes, to acknowledge and revel in other roles that you have in your life.

Do something just for yourself. If this feel selfish, take the following into consideration: leading a richer and fuller life will allow you to provide better care to your loved one and avoid burn out. You have to take care of your own needs before you can take care of others.

Respite Care

According to the Merriam-Webster Dictionary, respite means, "A short period of rest or relief from something difficult or unpleasant." Respite care is usually provided by someone who comes to stay with your loved one for a few hours so you can take a break. A respite caregiver might read your dad the newspaper or fix a simple lunch.

There are many potential sources of free or low-cost respite care: Family members, friends, neighbors, church members, and volunteers from social service agencies. In fact, the hardest part about finding respite care is steeling your nerve and asking for it. So many caregivers "don't want to impose" or "would hate to have someone feeling like they had to help me."

The truth is that the important people in your life probably want to help you. They just don't know how. So, the next time somebody says, "Call me if I can help," take a deep breath and say, "I have some errands to run Friday morning. Could you come over and sit with Dad for a couple of hours?"

If the first person you ask says no, ask again. And again. Ask your clergy to put an announcement in the church bulletin that you're looking for helpers. Call agencies that deal with your loved one's injury or disease and ask if they are aware of any resources for volunteer or low-cost respite care in the community.

If you're too shy to make these requests yourself, track down an outgoing friend or family member who has offered to help and say something like, "I need you to make some phone calls for me. Can you find a few people who would be willing to stay with Dad a few hours every week?"

Private Duty Care

Private duty workers usually have training and experience with senior in-home care. They can usually help with all aspects of care from transferring, dressing, bathing, and toileting to meal preparation, mental stimulation and transportation.

While caregivers can be hired through a job listing or the Internet, there are several pitfalls to this scenario. Hiring a worker privately means you are responsible to do background checks and to report what you pay the worker to the IRS for tax purposes, since he or she would be your private employee. There is no company insurance to rely on in the unfortunate case of damage to the home or financial abuse and a no-show from an unreliable caregiver means your loved one will be alone for an indefinite period of time.

Home care agencies also provide private duty care and reputable agencies have high-caliber caregiver employees who make all the difference to patients and their families. Agency caregivers are usually insured and bonded, which means there is the peace of mind associated with insurance coverage. They have also been through thorough background checks and all payment issues including taxes are addressed through the agency. Furthermore, if you don't like the first caregiver the agency assigns you, you can request another one. If one caregiver is unable to come to work on a day when you need her, the agency will have back-up caregivers that can be assigned on short notice.

There are some programs (such as the VA) that can help pay for the cost of agency care. And most long-term care insurance policies will pay for in-home private duty care. Depending on where you live, your local senior services program may be able to cover the cost of a few hours of private duty care each week. If your loved one has few assets and little income, they can apply for the state's Medicaid program in the United States, and there are equivalent programs in Canada and other countries. Once approved for Medicaid, you can inquire about a program called Home and Community Based Services (HCBS). Through this program Medicaid pays for a few hours of private duty care in the home every week. Medicare, unfortunately, does not pay for any private duty care.

Home Healthcare

Home healthcare is a skilled service covered by Medicare Part A and various private insurance companies. It is tailored for people who are home bound and who require the service of a nurse or a physical, occupational, or speech therapist. While your loved one is on home healthcare, a home health aide may be assigned to help with personal care. Unlike respite care and private duty care, which you can arrange yourself, home healthcare must be ordered by a doctor.

Reasons why a doctor might order home healthcare include wounds (such as bedsores), an unstable medical condition that requires monitoring, a need for IV drugs, a need for rehabilitation services to return your loved one to a prior level of functioning, or a new diagnosis or treatment that you and the patient must learn to manage.

Medicare paid home healthcare typically only lasts a few weeks or a few months, but it is a great alternative to trying to get your loved one out to see the doctor. Once the home healthcare period is over, you might consider hiring a private duty home care agency to continue to offer care.

Hospice

Hospice care is appropriate if your loved one has a life-limiting illness that is expected to result in death in six months or less, and if they have stopped all curative treatment for the illness. Like home healthcare, hospice care must be ordered by a physician. The hospice care involves a case manager who coordinates the care with you, the patient, the patient's doctor, and the rest of the hospice team. Other team members might include an LPN or LVN, a hospice aide to help with personal care, a medical social worker to assist with emotional support and community resources, a nondenominational chaplain for spiritual support, and a volunteer who can help with respite care.

The goal of hospice is to manage symptoms and help the individual live the last months as fully as possible. A person on hospice does not have to be home bound and if they feel well enough, they are encouraged to get out and do the things they enjoy.

After six months on hospice care, the individual is again assessed by a doctor. If the doctor finds that a terminal illness still exists and the person is declining, he can remain on hospice care. If, as sometimes happens, the disease process has slowed or stopped and the person is no longer declining—or is seven doing better—he must be discharged from hospice. He can be readmitted if the disease process becomes active again.

Medicare Part A covers all the costs of hospice care. Most private insurance companies also offer hospice benefits. If your loved one qualifies for hospice but doesn't have insurance, ask your doctor if there are any local not-for-profit hospice organizations that will treat people with no payor source.

Support Groups

Asked if she had any special advice for family caregivers, Emily Mangini, Care Manager at Home Care Assistance in Palo Alto, California, replied immediately, "Get involved in a support group." A support group is a group of people who are going through the same type of thing you are although, of course, no two caregiving situations are exactly alike. Support group members can cheer your successes, offer words of comfort when things aren't going well, and sometimes provide valuable advice about caregiving techniques that worked for their loved one.

Finding a support group that fits into your schedule usually takes a few phone calls. A good place to start is the local chapter of any organization that addresses your loved one's illness. For instance, if your loved one has Alzheimer's or a related type of dementia, you might want to call the local chapter of the Alzheimer's Association and ask about their support group schedule.

If that doesn't help, try calling your church, a local hospital or nursing facility and ask if they are aware of any support groups for caregivers. If you can't find anything that meets your needs in your community, consider joining an online forum or chat room for caregivers. One excellent site that offers terrific information and online support groups for caregivers is called simply Caregiving (http://www.caregiving.com/). Another place to try is the Caregivers Discussions form at Cancer Compass (http://www.cancercompass.com/message-board/caregivers/1,0,122.htm).

EIGHT

How to Do a Transfer

A transfer is simply helping a person move from one position to another. Moving between a bed and a wheelchair is a transfer. So is moving between a wheelchair and a commode, or from one bed to another. There are many different methods available to help transfer your loved one. This chapter examines the most common methods.

Stand-By Assist

Stand-by assist requires relatively little of the caregiver. It is a technique used with people who are still able to move around fairly independently but who are sometimes unsteady on their feet when getting up. The help required in a stand-by assist usually involves preparing required equipment, providing verbal cues, and offering light physical assistance. For instance, if you want to transfer your loved one from the bed to a bedside commode, get the bedside commode, make sure the lid is raised, and place the commode at a 90-degree angle to the bed.

Next, tell the person what you want him to do. “I’m going to help you to the commode, Dad, and I need you to sit up on the side of your bed.” Offer an arm or take his hands and gently draw him forwards if he needs your support sitting up.

Check to make sure he is wearing footwear with non-skid soles. Transferring a person who is barefoot or wearing only socks increases the risk of slipping and falling. Remind the person to sit forward on the bed and put both feet firmly on the floor. Then say, "At the count of three, I want you to stand up." Again, be ready to provide light physical assistance if he has trouble getting to his feet. Once he is standing, give the next verbal instruction. "Turn so that you're facing me." Guide him in making the turn if necessary. Line him up with the commode so that all he has to do is sit down. "You're right behind the commode. All you have to do is sit down." If he has trouble, guide his hands to the railings on the commode for balance.

The stand-by assist is the least strenuous transfer for both you and your loved one. You should use it as long as the person is able to sit up, stand, turn, and sit back down again with minimal assistance.

Pivot Transfer

The pivot transfer uses the same basic idea as the stand-by assist, but it requires you to do more physical lifting. For example, suppose you are going to help your father transfer from his bed to a wheelchair. Again, prepare the environment by bringing the wheelchair into the room and place it at a 90-degree angle, facing the foot of the bed. Swing back or remove the leg rests so your father will not trip over them.

If your father cannot sit up without assistance, tell him that you are going to help him sit on the edge of the bed. Stand sideways facing the foot of the bed and slip your left forearm beneath his shoulders and your right arm under his knees. Using your legs, lift and turn him so that his legs are hanging over the bed and his shoulders are elevated. Maneuver him into a seated position. If he cannot maintain this position on his own, you may need to prop him up with pillows.

Next, place a gait belt around his waist. It is much safer for him and for you if you use a gait belt to assist with transfers and not try to move him by pulling on his arms. Check his footgear and make sure he is wearing shoes or slippers with non-skid soles. Place his feet flat on the floor.

Then stand directly in front of him, using your knees as added support. Some caregivers are more comfortable with a knee-to-knee position. Others prefer to have the person's knees between their own knees.

Move close to your father, bend your knees, grasp the gait belt from behind, and tell him to push down with his feet on the count of three. On the count of three, as he pushes down with his feet, you pull up on the gait belt. Use your legs to do the lifting. When you are standing face to face, use the gait belt to pivot both your body and his, encouraging him to help you as much as possible. Make sure he is aligned with the chair and then gently lower him onto the seat of the chair. Replace the footrests, offer him a blanket to wrap around his shoulders or put on his lap, and help prop him up with pillows and cushions if necessary.

Standing Assist Devices

Pivot transfers will generally work as long as your loved one is still able to support some of his own weight. If your loved one is much larger than you or can only support his weight for a short time, you might have to use a mechanical device.

A standing assist device is used for seniors who still have some ability to bear weight. The hardware includes two wheeled legs, a plastic platform to support the feet and knees, handrails, a hook, and a pneumatic lift device. The software includes a vest or belt that is placed around the back and attached to the hook.

After helping your loved one sit on the side of the bed as described in the pivot transfer, place the vest or belt around shoulders and back. Attach the vest to the hook. Check for proper footgear and then have the person place his feet on the platform and his hands on the handrails.

Assume that you are going to start pulling him into a standing position. Engage the pneumatic device, which will lift him to a standing position. Ideally, the person is supported by his own calves, the handrails, and the vest around his back. While your loved one is standing, you can clean them and put fresh adult briefs on if necessary. Then role the device to the commode, wheelchair, or wherever the person will be sitting. Letting him know what you are going to do, gently lower him into the seat. Provide pillows, cushions, blankets, etc. to make sure he is comfortable. Whenever you use a standing assist device, make sure the person really is able to bear at least some weight. Otherwise, the device could strain their back and shoulders.

The Hoyer Lift

A Hoyer lift is another type of mechanical lift. It is used for people who cannot bear any weight on their own. The Hoyer lift hardware consists of two legs on wheels. The legs are parallel to each other but can be moved apart to maneuver a person into a wheelchair. The Hoyer also features a large hook, a pneumatic lifting device and a sling with six straps.

To place the sling underneath your loved one, ask him to roll so that he is facing away from you. If he cannot roll by himself, come around to the side of the bed that you want him to face, put your hands on his shoulders and knees, and roll him towards you. You may have to arrange pillows behind his back and knees so that he does not simply roll back the other way. Go back to the other side of the bed, roll the sling in half, and push the side you have rolled up as far underneath the body as you can reach. Then remove the pillows keeping him in place. Help him roll towards you and replace the positioning pillows. Go around to the other side of the bed, find the edge of the rolled up sling and pull it through. Then allow him to rest on his back again. The centerline of the sling and the backbone of your loved one should be aligned.

The person is now lying on top of the sling. Three of the straps should be on the right and three of the straps should be on his left. They should be located roughly at leg, waist, and shoulder level. Pull the straps at leg level between the legs. Then attach all of the straps to the hook. Tell your loved one that you are getting ready to lift him and engage the pneumatic device. If he appears frightened, reassure him that he is safe and that you will have him comfortable in his wheelchair in just a moment. When he is suspended, position the lift over the wheelchair and slowly lower the sling into the chair. The sling will remain beneath your loved one as long as he is sitting up.

Hoyer lifts can help give mobility to people who would not otherwise have it, but they should be used with caution. When used on carpet, Hoyer lifts can tip if they are not balanced correctly. If the person being transferred exceeds the recommended maximum weight, a Hoyer lift is not safe. That is why some facilities have a rule that a Hoyer lift cannot be used by a single caregiver. In these cases, two or more caregivers must be involved when a Hoyer lift is used. Although it is not always feasible to have two caregivers in a home care setting, two people can make a Hoyer lift transfer go much more smoothly.

Draw Sheet Transfer

A draw sheet transfer is used when a person who is lying on his back needs to be transferred from bed to bed or from bed to gurney. A draw sheet is simply a thick bed sheet that is used to bear the weight during the transfer. A draw sheet transfer requires two caregivers, one on each side. It works better with the use of friction-reducing surfaces such as sliding boards, decreased friction mattress covers, or, in a pinch, large plastic bags. The two surfaces should be as close to equal height as possible.

To place the draw sheet, caregivers assist the person with rolling onto his side. They then place the folded draw sheet under the back and hips. The person is then assisted to roll onto the other side and the caregiver unrolls the draw sheet. When the person is returned to lying on his back, he should be lying roughly in the middle of the draw sheet. To transfer, each caregiver stands on one side of the bed and grips the draw sheet in the middle. After explaining what will happen, one caregiver counts to three, and together the caregivers slide the person from one surface to the other. Draw sheet transfers may be used to place a person on a gurney for a trip to the emergency room or to transfer him back to bed upon his return.

NINE

How to Give a Bath

In addition to daily hygiene care, most seniors need a full bath at least twice a week, unless the doctor tells you otherwise. Bathing can be awkward and embarrassing for some caregivers. It is important to communicate openly and honestly with your loved one and try to find solutions for difficult moments. Give the person you are caring for as much say as possible in the proceedings and encourage them to do everything possible for themselves.

Supplies

Nothing is more annoying than being cold and wet and having your caregiver run in and out of the bathroom or the bedroom looking for supplies. Therefore, you should gather everything you will need before the bath. If the person will be washing in the tub or shower, you will probably need soap or a soapless skin cleanser (which is gentler on dry skin), lotions or creams to act as a moisture barrier and protect the skin, baby powder to ease friction in spots where the skin rubs together, antiperspirants or deodorants, wash cloths, warm towels, bath blankets, and clean clothes or a gown to change into after the bath.

Stand-By Bathing Assist

As in transferring, you may be required to do little more than provide verbal cues and minor physical assistance. Make sure that you are on hand when your loved one gets into and out of the tub or shower. If they complain of weakness while in the shower, consider installing a tub bench. These benches are available at most pharmacies and discount stores. Handrails should also be mounted securely in the tub or shower.

Once safely in the tub or shower, let your loved one do most of the washing. Offer to wash difficult-to-reach places, like the back. As you assist in and out of the tub or shower, pat the skin dry with a towel and take a look to make sure it really is clean. If you find an area that didn't get washed, say something neutral like, "Whoops, that spot got missed. Let me take care of it for you." Once your loved one is clean and dry, help him change into a fresh hospital gown or clothing.

Full Assistance with Shower or Tub Bath

Your loved one may be too tired or suffer from too many coordination problems to bathe themselves. In this case, you will be responsible for giving all or most of the bath. Begin by gathering all of the required supplies, as mentioned above.

Announce that it's time for the weekly bath. Many people get cold while bathing or dislike the feeling of being undressed in front of a family member, close friend, or caregiver. People with dementia may insist that they have already had a bath that day. Be sympathetic, but firm. "I know you don't like it, but it will only take a few minutes." Or "Just think how beautiful and fresh you'll look when we're all finished."

Once inside the bathroom, place a nonskid mat in the tub. Put a tub bench on top of the mat. Start the water, checking the temperature frequently. Help your loved one undress and get into the tub. It may be easier to sit on the edge of the tub.

Then you can gently swing his legs into the tub and help slide him over to the bench. They may need to rest a few minutes to start bathing after the ordeal of getting into the bathtub.

When your loved one is ready to start bathing, encourage him to do as much as possible for himself. The areas of the body that need to be washed include the head, neck, and face, the chest and abdomen, the genital area, the arms and legs, and the back and buttocks. You will probably need to help with the back and buttocks. Be matter-of-fact as you go about the task of bathing and use long, firm strokes.

Talking about something that interests you during the bath may help distract you from any embarrassment you might feel. You may also play your loved one's favorite music to reassure and soothe him. When you have finished washing the body, ask if he would like his hair washed. Don't make a big deal out of it if he refuses. It can always be done on another day.

Before assisting your loved one out of the tub, make sure that all soap has been rinsed off. Soap left behind will dry the skin. Your loved one should exit the tub or shower very carefully, as his feet will be wet and slippery. Remember to have slippers with non-skid soles ready as soon as the bath or shower is complete.

Once out of the shower, drape bath blankets around him for modesty and then pat—do not rub—dry with warm towels. Finally, apply lotion, powder, deodorant, and cologne as preferred. Make sure to dress him in clean clothes.

Full Assistance with Bed Bath

If the older adult is confined to bed, you will need to give him a bed bath. In addition to the supplies that you need for a tub bath, you will also need bed protectors to keep the bed linens from getting wet, a wash basin with warm (not hot) water, and clean linens. Place the basin, washcloths, and towels on the bedside table. As with any other procedure, explain exactly what you are going to do. Reassure him that he will feel much more comfortable and clean and that he will look much better. Ask if he would like the television or a CD of favorite music playing during the bath.

When you have put your loved one at ease as much as possible, remove the bedspread and the blankets from the bed. Fold them and put them aside. Place the bath blanket over the linens. Help the person undress, keeping their modesty intact as much as possible. Unless you are caring for a person who requires that the head of the bed be elevated, lay the bed as flat as possible. Place a towel over the chest, then dip a wash cloth into the basin of warm water and gently wash the face and neck. Remember to wash behind the ears, at the corners of the eyes, and at the collarbone where sweat often accumulates. If you are using soap, rinse the skin clean and pat the face dry.

Put the bed protector under the arm to keep the blankets dry. Then draw one arm out from under the bath sheet. Wash in long strokes from the shoulder to the fingertips. Then lift the arm so you can wash underneath. Rinse away the soap, pat that arm dry with a towel, cover the arm with the bath blanket, expose the other arm and wash it in the same way.

Next, place a towel over the chest, under the bath blanket. Fold the bath blanket down to about the level of the waist and wash the chest. When patting a woman's chest dry with a towel, be sure to dry the areas under the breasts where skin touches skin. Now fold the bath blanket down to the hips and wash the abdomen. If your loved one is heavy-set, make sure to pat the folds of skin dry.

Pull the bath blanket back up and remove the towel from the chest. At this point, you might want to get fresh warm water in the basin. Then remove the bath blanket from the leg and wash the leg with long, firm strokes. When you have finished, set the basin on the bed protector and place the entire foot inside the basin. Wash the entire foot, including the area between the toes, and dry it carefully with a towel. Do the same thing with the other leg and the other foot.

Then take a minute to change the water in the basin again. Help your loved one turn on her side so she is facing away from you. Lift the bed blanket to expose the back and buttocks and put your bed protector along the person's back. Starting at the top of the back, wash the back and buttocks and pat dry.

If your loved one is physically and cognitively able to do so, encourage him to wash the genital area while you step outside. If he is not capable of managing this part of his care, gently wash the genital area and pat it dry. Cover the person up with the bath blanket.

Put lotion, powder, deodorant, and cologne on the skin. Then help the person into new clothing. If the bed linens were wet or soiled during the process of bathing, change them. Remove all the soiled linens and the bathing equipment so that the room looks fresh and clean.

Bag Baths

Bag baths provide an alternative to full baths. A bag bath is a plastic bag containing several disposable washcloths that have been soaked in a soapless cleanser. The bag is placed in the microwave for a few minutes to warm the cloths. Then each cloth is used to clean a different body part. At the end of the bath, simply dispose of the bag baths. The whole procedure takes only a few minutes and many seniors prefer it to the trauma of getting into a bathtub and having each part of their body washed and rinsed.

Hair Care

Hair is one of the physical attributes that we use to express our personality and style. Try to respect your loved one's style and preferences where hair is concerned. For instance, if your Mom is proud of her long, wavy hair, don't insist that she cut it just because a short hairstyle would be easier to care for.

Washing Hair

As people get older, their joints may become stiff. Some find it difficult or painful to raise their hands up to their heads for any length of time. This means you may need to help with hair washing. Nobody likes the feeling of having greasy, dirty hair, so wash your loved one's hair at least once or twice a week.

If they are still able to get into the shower or tub and sit on a tub bench, wash their hair while in the shower. Use a small amount of a mild shampoo and lather it throughout the hair. You can also provide a gentle, soothing scalp massage. For rinsing, consider purchasing and installing a handheld showerhead. They cost approximately $30 to $50 and are available at hardware stores.

They make rinsing your loved one's hair a snap. Thorough rinsing is an important part of hair washing. If you've ever had to rush through your morning shower and gone through the day with dry shampoo in your hair, you know that it isn't the least bit pleasant or comfortable.

If your loved one is bedbound, you have two options. One is to purchase an inflatable shampoo trough, available through most pharmacies and medical supply companies. The bedbound person's head rests in the trough, which catches water and shampoo and keeps the bed from getting wet. Place a wash cloth over your loved one's eyes to keep out shampoo. If your loved one is able, ask him to hold it in place. Then pour warm water from a pitcher over your loved one's hair. Once his hair is moist, apply the shampoo and massage it into the hair and scalp. Carefully rinse your loved one's hair with more warm water from the pitcher. After the shampoo is completed, empty the contents of the trough into a basin and dispose of it. Whenever you give your loved one a shampoo, make sure to wrap his head in a soft, warm towel so that he doesn't become chilled.

Another option for cleansing the hair and scalp of a bedbound senior is to use a dry or "rinse-less" shampoo, available at most pharmacies. Some people love these shampoos for their ease of use. Others complain that rinse-less shampoos leave residue in the hair and cause itching and scalp irritation. Let your loved one select the method of hair care that they prefer.

Hair Styling

Your loved one will need regular haircuts. They may also want to get their hair curled, permed, or colored. If an older adult is able to leave the home at all, he may enjoy a trip to the barbershop or beauty salon. If your loved one cannot leave the home, you may be able to find someone who is willing to make home visits for an occasional haircut. If you have a family member, friend, or neighbor who is a hair stylist, see if that person would be willing to help out for a little extra money. You may also want to ask your loved one's current stylist if they would be willing to make a home visit from time to time. If you're having trouble finding someone, call a few local beauty schools to see if any of their students might be interested in helping your loved one. Of course, if you feel comfortable with your own abilities as a hair stylist, you can take on this job for yourself.

Now that you know how to keep your loved one feeling clean and refreshed on the outside, it's time to turn our attention to food and nutrition. What your loved one eats can make a difference in how he feels, physically and emotionally.

TEN

How to Feed Home Bound Seniors

According to the New Food Pyramid released by the U.S. Department of Agriculture in 2005, the general adult population should eat five to six servings of grain each day. Three of those servings should be whole grains. The pyramid also suggests a wide spectrum of vegetables and fruits, a limited amount of vegetable oils, three or more servings of low-fat, calcium rich foods, and about five ounces of lean protein. Of course, that same pyramid also suggests that adults be physically active thirty minutes a day, a rare feat for most older adults.

When you think about the government recommended diet, along with the way many seniors eat, it is apparent that many are nutritionally at risk, and thus may need to alter their food intake. According to Glenda Kindler, nutrition specialist at University of Missouri, some of the factors that affect seniors' nutrition include an inability to shop and cook for themselves, a tendency to eat alone, use of multiple medications that affect the appetite in various ways, loss of appetite due to physical health or depression, and nutritional concerns unique to many disease processes.

In an ideal world, every senior should ask for input on diet from both a physician and a nutritionist. From there, the physician should arrange for the nutritionist to visit the home and make recommendations. In reality, however, nutrition consultations are seldom obtained for seniors.

That is why we published our companion volume (*Happy To 102! The Best Kept Secrets To A Long And Happy Life, Home Care Assistance, 2007*) to describe the Balanced Care Method of home care, which includes a Balanced Care diet recommendation for seniors at home. Please consult it for a detailed overview of the power of an appropriate diet for healthy longevity.

Always be aware that appetite decreases with illness and inactivity. *Happy to 102!* suggests that caregivers offer several small snacks during the day as opposed to three heavy meals that may seem overwhelming. Caregivers should focus on protein (preferably fish-based) to keep the skin and nails healthy. Balanced Care also recommends a diet high in fiber to keep the bowels moving. Older adults tend to get little exercise and, thus, are more likely to become constipated. Balance Care reminds caregivers to offer fluids frequently to avoid dehydration and urinary problems. Finally, we recommend frequent snacks consisting of fruit and nuts.

If the person you are taking care of is still able to make choices about what he likes to eat, offer him options. "It's lunchtime, Dad. I could warm up the rest of the chicken and we have blueberries for desert." When you serve the food, make it as attractive as possible. Vary color and texture and consider using plates and glasses with interesting designs.

Feeding

If your loved one is able to eat on his own, by all means encourage him to do so. In fact, do everything you can to extend this behavior. For instance, when your loved one is no longer able to easily use utensils, try finger foods instead.

There will probably come a time, however, when you are responsible for feeding your loved one. If necessary, use a wheelchair for meals. If your loved one is bedbound, make sure the head of the bed is elevated as much as can be tolerated. Never try to give a person food or fluids while he is lying flat on his back, as he is likely to choke.

When you are ready to start feeding, place a napkin around the neck so clothes don't get soiled. Have a warm washcloth on hand to wipe up spills and saliva. Set the plate of food down in front of your loved one. If he doesn't see well or if he has severe cognitive problems, say out loud what is on the plate.

Before you place a bite of food in your loved one's mouth, say what they will be eating. "Here's a spoonful of beans, Mom." If your loved one has dementia, watch closely to make sure that he chews and swallows. People with end-stage dementia may forget what to do with food, "pocketing" it in the side of their mouths. They may also try to spit food out, especially if they don't like the taste. Provide gentle verbal cues, like, "Chew and swallow." Offer your loved one a sip of water between bites to make sure the mouth is clear. Do not offer the second bite until he has swallowed the first bite. Also, do not mix different foods together unless you know your loved one likes them that way.

Make mealtime as pleasant and unhurried as possible. While you are waiting for your loved one to get ready for the next bite, talk about something interesting that has happened during your day or something funny that a grandchild did. Some people enjoy listening to music or watching TV during meals.

Once your loved one has finished eating, provide oral care. Encourage sitting after the meal with a brief chat. This will aid digestion and decrease the likelihood of acid reflux.

Texture

Depending on your loved one's condition, they may have trouble swallowing certain types of food. For example, people who have had a stroke may choke on solid foods. People with end-stage Alzheimer's may not be able to drink liquids without aspirating them, pulling them into the lungs where they can cause infections such as pneumonia.

Even if your loved one is still relatively independent with eating, try to share at least one meal a day with them. Watch for symptoms like gasping, coughing, or choking with swallowing. Keep track of which foods and fluids your loved one seems to tolerate well and which foods and fluids cause coughing.

Call your loved one's doctor with your observations. The doctor might want to arrange a test called a swallow study or a speech therapy consult. Speech therapists can sometimes work with clients who are having trouble swallowing food and teach them new ways to position their heads, such as tucking the chin, that make swallowing easier.

Other times, however, a physical therapist will be unable to resolve the problem and will recommend a change in the texture of the diet. This will probably involve switching your loved one to soft or pureed foods, and perhaps thickened liquids as well.

Liquids are thickened by adding a stiffening powder to regular fluids. The powder gives the liquid a syrupy or honey-like texture. Some people don't like this new texture or complain that the powder has an odd taste. They may become resistive to drinking any liquid that is thickened.

The family and the individual now have a decision to make. Is it better to let the people enjoy drinking regular fluids and risk aspiration pneumonia? Or is it better to give the fluids that your loved one doesn't like to decrease the risk of aspirating?

Jayne Ichban, C.N.A., Care Manager, Home Care Assistance in Los Gatos, California, shares her experiences with Gladys, an 89-year-old woman. Although Gladys had mild cognitive impairment, she was still able to understand consequences and make decisions. She loved coffee more than anything else. When Gladys had a stroke and the doctor put her on a thickened-liquid diet, she was miserable. Gladys spent most of her days trying to coax her caregivers into giving her a "regular" cup of coffee.

This woman's physician said she could go back to drinking the coffee she loved but it might lead to pneumonia and shorten her life. On the other hand, if she drank thickened liquids, she could probably live for several more years. Jayne remembers, "It didn't take Gladys two minutes to make her choice. We all laughed when she said, 'Years of this hell? Why would I want that?'"

With her family and physician in full agreement, Gladys was free to have her coffee again. She survived three more months before she developed aspiration pneumonia and passed away in her sleep. When Jayne asked Gladys' daughter if she was comfortable with the decision her mother had made, the daughter replied, "Absolutely, yes. She lived and died the way she wanted."

Feeding Tubes

If your loved one is unable to take enough nourishment to sustain life by mouth, doctors will place a feeding tube that goes directly into the stomach. Tubes intended for short-term use are usually inserted through the nostrils. However, if it becomes clear that the individual will continue to need nourishment by tube for a significant amount of time, the care team may surgically insert a feeding tube into the stomach through the abdominal wall. This is called a percutaneous endoscopic gastrostomy, or PEG tube. The PEG tube is designed so that it cannot be pulled out by accident. Two to three inches of tubing extend from the incision. This is where feedings are given.

Anyone who has a PEG tube placed in their stomach should have a consultation with a dietician before leaving the hospital. The dietician will recommend a brand of liquid to use for tube feedings. The dietician will also explain how many calories and fluids are needed and how much protein should be given each day.

Administering tube feedings can be a little intimidating at first but the procedure is not difficult once you get the hang of it. First, because you are working with an open incision (stoma), wash your hands carefully with soap and water and don gloves to avoid spreading infection. Next, prepare the formula as instructed by the dietician. Make sure that your loved one is sitting up at a 30-degree angle at minimum. This will help prevent regurgitation or aspiration of the food.

Next, take a moment to look at the tube. There should be a mark on the tube where it is supposed to enter the abdominal wall. If the tube is not placed properly or if it has come out, your loved one will have to go to the hospital immediately to have it replaced. Doctors can replace it through the original incision for the first 24 hours or so. After that, replacing the tube requires another surgical procedure.

If all is well, flush the tube with water at room temperature. Then, slowly administer the formula, also at room temperature. The formula must be administered very slowly to avoid causing your loved one uncomfortable symptoms, such as abdominal pain, diarrhea, nausea, vomiting, or distension of the stomach. A single feeding can take up to an hour.

Make the most of this time with your loved one. If he can talk, try to get him involved in a conversation. Even if he can't respond, you can still continue talking. Talk about your day, about anything going on in the news that might seem interesting, or about family memories. If you run out of things to say, watch a favorite television program together or listen to music that you both like. When you have finished administering the formula, flush the tube again with water to help prevent clogging.

Another option you might want to speak to your doctor about is continuous feeding. This involves connecting a feeding pump that slowly infuses food into the tube over a period of several hours. Another type of continuous feeding is called gravity feeding. The formula is prepared and hung in a bag over the feeding tube. Gravity will cause the formula to drip into the tube slowly over a period of four to six hours. Even if your loved one is receiving continuous feeding, you will still need to flush the tube with water every four to eight hours.

If, during or after feeding, your loved one complains of bloating, you can ease his discomfort by removing the feeding cap from the tube. This opens the PEG to air and the excess gas can be expelled from your loved one's stomach. Sometimes coughing helps decompress the stomach more quickly.

Nutritional Decisions and End of Life

Most people do not have a problem having the feeding tube placed in their stomach if the tube will provide the temporary nourishment they need to get them through a disease process. A person receiving rehabilitation services after a stroke is likely to come off the tube and eat orally again one day.

Maura Barilaro, RN, Director of Nursing for Home Care Assistance in the Washington DC region recalls a recent experience with a client who had suffered a stroke, which had resulted in a decrease in his swallowing ability. As a result, he got a PEG tube. He also received speech and swallow therapy while in rehab. His ability to swallow improved somewhat but he had a poor appetite and needed nutritional and fluid supplements via the tube.

He was discharged from the rehab facility and came home with the help of a live-in caregiver. As part of the discharge plan, the doctor's order was to give him one can of tube feeding supplement if he ate less that 50% of his meal. However, this gentleman preferred not to eat the traditional three big meals a day, but instead had five smaller meals each day. As a result, he always ate nearly 100% of each of the five meals. Therefore, he never needed the supplement via the PEG tube. The only requirement was a tube flush with water as needed. So, after two months of no supplemental feedings and no weight loss, the doctor removed the tube, much to the delight of the family.

Working under close supervision of Maura, the live-in caregivers were able to create a healthy diet that met all of his nutritional needs. This gentleman was able to thrive without the tube while enjoying a wide range of tastes and culinary experiences.

Nutritional Needs of the Dying

As people reach the end of a terminal illness and begin the process known as "active dying," their nutritional needs change. The body is shutting down. The stomach no longer needs food, nor even knows what to do with it. Artificial feeding usually results in vomiting, diarrhea, and uncomfortable cramping. Instead of keeping the person's body healthy and hydrated, fluids pool under—and often weep through—the skin.

These are very difficult realizations for family members of the dying person. Food may be equated with love and nurturing. So it seems counter-intuitive to stop "nurturing" a loved one at this point.

You can still, however, offer both nurturing and comfort without overloading your loved one's dying system. First, according to hospice nurse Barbara Karnes in her book, *Gone from my Sight*, the dying person's main needs are emotional and spiritual rather than nutritional. Sit quietly by your loved one, hold his hand, and tell him that you love him.

Second, if your loved one's lips look dry and parched, apply a lip balm, or place a wash cloth soaked in cool water on your loved one's lips. To keep the inside of the mouth feeling fresh, use a moist toothette, a small sponge attached to the end of a stick about the length of a lollypop, to swab your loved one's mouth. Don't forget to swab the roof of the mouth or the area under the tongue. A small amount of crushed ice is also beneficial to keep the inside of the mouth fresh.

Finally, never place food or fluid in the mouth of an unconscious, comatose, or sleeping person. You will only cause choking. If the person does wake up and asks for a special food or liquid, provide it. They will probably only want to take a couple of bites before drifting back to sleep. Usually, people stop eating and drinking entirely a day or two before they pass away. Their bodies no longer need the sustenance, and medications are given to control any discomfort that might exist. Accept this as normal and as part of the process of dying.

The next chapter discusses how oral care and the proper techniques for keeping teeth and gums healthy.

ELEVEN

How to Care for Teeth and Gums

We all know that poor oral care can lead to unpleasant conditions such as bad breath, gum disease and, for people who still have their own teeth, painful cavities. What is not common knowledge is that some studies have shown that good oral care in seniors might actually reduce the risk of respiratory infections and a host of other diseases.

The groundswell of evidence linking poor oral health with systemic diseases, including cardiovascular disease, diabetes, and respiratory problems, has prompted the world's most prestigious healthcare institutions to place a renewed focus on good oral healthcare as a preventive measure.

"I've seen seniors who haven't been able to leave their homes for years due to aging and mobility issues or, in some cases, agoraphobia. As all the research continues to point to the significant links between oral healthcare and overall health, it's becoming even more important that home-bound seniors receive proper dental care," shared Dr. Amir Ghorbani, Founder and Primary Care Dentist of Home Care Dentist.

Daily brushing and flossing are crucial activities that affect our health, and seniors need dental care every day, too. In fact, dental care is just as important to a senior's health and daily routine as taking medications and getting physical exercise. A healthy mouth helps seniors to eat well, avoid pain and tooth loss, and maintain a positive outlook on life.

Natural Teeth

If the senior has natural teeth, he can use a toothbrush or an electric toothbrush with soft bristles and a choice of fluoride-based toothpaste to brush his teeth. Using mouthwash after brushing leaves a fresh taste in the mouth and reduces the growth of bacteria that can cause cavities. Chlorhexidine rinses fight germs that cause gum disease. You should also encourage your loved one to use dental floss once a day.

Most people are able to provide at least some oral care for themselves. If your loved one cannot stand for long, you may need to assist. The National Institute of Dental and Craniofacial Research and Dr. Ghorbani of Home Care Dentist offer the following tips to handle any anxiety on the part of the senior:

- At first, dental care can be frightening to some people. Try the "**tell-show-do**" approach to deal with this natural reaction. **Tell** the senior about each step before you do it. For example, explain how you'll help him or her brush and what it feels like. **Show** how you're going to do each step before you do it. Also, it might help to let the senior hold and feel the toothbrush and floss. **Do** the steps in the same way that you've explained them.

- Offer dental care in an environment that is most comfortable for the person. In some cases, this may not be the bathroom and may instead be the living room, a bedroom, or the kitchen. Any clean space can be made appropriate for the hygiene session, as long as there is good light and a table on which you can place the necessary supplies, including the toothbrush, toothpaste, a bowl, and a cup of water.

- Give the senior time to adjust to dental care. Be patient as that person learns to trust you working in and around his or her mouth. This may mean taking breaks between quadrants of the mouth.

- Use your voice and body to communicate that you care. Give positive feedback often to reinforce good behavior.

- Have a routine for dental care. Use the same technique at the same time and place every day. A routine might soothe fears or help eliminate some of the anxiety associated with the oral health process.

- Be creative. Some caregivers allow those they care for to hold a favorite toy or special item for comfort. Others make dental care a game or play a person's favorite music.

If your loved one is not able to brush their own teeth, you can assist by moistening the toothbrush and squeezing a pea-size amount of toothpaste onto the bristles. Tell your loved one what you are about to do and be as gentle as possible. Seniors who are confused as a result of dementia may be especially resistive to dental care, because it is not pleasant to have what is seemingly a strange object placed into the mouth.

Start brushing the outer surface of the top teeth. Brushing in a circular motion, start at the back of the mouth and work your way around to the front teeth and then the teeth on the other side. Do the same thing with the bottom teeth. Take some time and allow the person to rinse his mouth out if needed.

Next, ask your loved one to open his mouth a little wider and brush the inner surface of the top and bottom teeth. Again, allow time to rinse and spit. Finally, brush the chewing surfaces of the teeth and the tongue. Provide water and a basin so that the person can rinse out all of the toothpaste. Consider using a finger wrapped in gauze to sweep the mouth if you suspect that the mouth was not rinsed fully. Use a washcloth to wipe away any toothpaste or water left on the face.

Next, cut a length of dental floss about 18 inches long. Wrap it around one finger of each hand. Starting with the back, upper teeth, insert the dental floss between two teeth, move it up and down gently, being careful not to injure the gums. Withdraw the dental floss from the mouth, adjust it so that a fresh bit of floss is available, and insert it between the next two teeth.

When you have finished flossing, have your loved one rinse again and pat the face dry with a washcloth. Finally, ask your loved one if they would like to rinse with mouthwash and assist in doing so. End the oral care by providing a moistening agent to the lips.

If your loved one cannot hold his mouth open, raise the head of the bed as tolerated and use a tongue depressor wrapped with gauze to hold the mouth open. Brush the teeth gently as described above. You will need to dip the toothbrush in water to help clear the mouth of toothpaste. Because of the risk of choking, do not use too much water and do not pour mouthwash into the mouth.

Keep in mind that toothbrushes typically need to be replaced every three months or after any contagious illness. For older adults, toothbrushes with soft bristles are best. Electric toothbrushes are a good option for those seniors with dexterity issues. If your loved one has a pacemaker, consult with a dentist about electric toothbrushes that will not interfere with the pacemaker's functionality.

No Teeth

Even a person with few or no teeth needs oral care. This can be provided with a toothette, a small sponge attached to a stick. Soak the toothette in water or mouthwash, as the individual prefers, and have him run it over his gums, tongue, and the insides of the cheeks.

Denture Care

Many people prefer to care for their own dentures. Depending on the person's mobility, you may need to provide some of the supplies, help with brushing or rinsing the dentures, or placing them in the denture cup. If your loved one is confused, one problem that may occur frequently is lost or missing dentures. Sometimes this occurs when the person tries to clean the dentures in the sink.

At other times, dentures may become uncomfortable and the person will take them out and "hide" them. It is not unusual to find dentures wrapped up in napkins and left on a dinner plate, in the trashcan, in the toilet, or even in the glasses case. If the person you are caring for cannot assist in denture care, you can clean his dentures. Assist with removing the dentures. Then take the dentures to a clean sink. You can use a special brush and cleanser made for dentures, or you may use a regular toothbrush and toothpaste as you and your loved one prefer.

Partially fill the sink with water, but do not place the dentures in the sink. Instead, wet the toothbrush and put some denture cleaner or toothpaste on it. Then hold the upper denture in one hand and carefully brush it until each surface is clean. Rinse it under running water and place it in the denture cup. Repeat the same process with the lower denture.

If the dentures are to be left out for a while, fill the denture cup with a mixture of water and mouthwash, place the dentures in the cup, and put the lid on the cup. Be sure to put the cup somewhere where you can find it easily and where it cannot accidentally be thrown away.

If the dentures are to be reinserted, help your loved one clean out the inside of their mouth with a soft-bristled toothbrush or a toothette, carefully reinsert the dentures, wipe any moisture from the person's mouth or face, and end the oral care by applying lip balm.

Oftentimes, the loss of appetite associated with aging is actually related to ill-fitting dentures. Dr. Ghorbani explains, "Teeth shift even in geriatric patients, so partial dentures may stop fitting properly if they're not worn for continuous periods of time. Full dentures may also need to be relined because the supporting tissue in the mouth changes in shape. General dentists are trained to reline dentures so that they have better retention and cause less irritation in the mouth. Prosthodontists specialize in making dentures and can be consulted with any questions on denture creation and fit."

Dental Check-Ups

Dentists recommend that older adults receive dental cleanings and check-ups at least twice per year. This can often be a challenge for many seniors. If your loved one is able to get up and around in a wheelchair, you can probably find a wheelchair van service which will take them to the dentist's office.

Otherwise, contact your community's local dental society to find out if there are dentists or dental services that make house calls. Dr. Ghorbani explains, "We began making dentistry house calls in the San Francisco Bay Area because we saw a great need for this service among seniors with mobility issues. There are several house call dentistry providers who offer a similar service in other parts of the country and in Canada. Local dental societies, Alzheimer's Associations, and councils on aging should have information on their community resource directories."

It's also important to find a dentist who understands your loved one's physical or neurological limitations and is willing to work with them. Some dementia patients, for instance, may become angry and resistive in the dentist's office. Dentists who have experience working with people with Alzheimer's disease often recommend a mild sedative before any dental procedures.

No Dental Care Available

If there is simply no dentist available to your loved one, make it a point to look inside his mouth at least once a week, even if he is still responsible for his own oral care. Check for bad breath, swelling and bleeding around the gums, and teeth that are obviously cracked or damaged. Ask your loved one if he has any kind of oral pain. If serious problems do arise, your loved one may have to be transported to a hospital to see an oral surgeon. Otherwise, simply continue to make sure that your loved one gets good oral care.

Taking care of a senior requires patience and skill. As a caregiver, you know this well. It is both challenging and rewarding to provide quality oral hygiene for another person. It takes time, energy, planning and the ability to manage various physical or behavioral concerns. Even so, it is extremely important and crucial to the senior's overall health. Brushing and flossing every day and seeing a dentist regularly can make a big difference in the quality of life of the person you care for.

Now that you've mastered oral hygiene, you're ready to move on to the next chapter, which discusses a difficult subject for most family caregivers. It explains how to change diapers and catheters.

TWELVE

How to Change Diapers and Catheters

Many seniors have occasional trouble with bladder or bowel incontinence. Even though your loved one may want to wear incontinence products for reassurance, encourage him or her to keep using the bathroom as long as possible. There are two good reasons for this. First, urine and feces can be very hard on the skin and can increase the likelihood of pressure ulcers. Second, being able to use the toilet is a matter of dignity.

There are a number of ways to help your loved one remain continent as long as possible. Introduce a toileting schedule. Every couple of hours, assist your loved one to the bathroom, whether they feel the "urge" to go or not. This makes it less likely that they will surprised by a strong bladder spasm.

You can also buy equipment that makes using the toilet easier. Many seniors may have trouble squatting low enough to sit on the toilet. A toilet riser consists of a frame that fits over the toilet, sturdy handrails, and an opening that should be positioned directly over your toilet seat. Your loved one can then sit on the riser and not have to worry about getting up and down.

Another valuable piece of equipment is a bedside commode. If your loved one moves slowly or has very intense urges to urinate or defecate, having a commode in the same room may mean the difference between making it to the bathroom on time and having an accident. A commode is composed of a sturdy frame with handrails on each side and a round opening in the center. Beneath the opening is a bucket to catch urine and feces. The opening has a lid, so that if your loved one uses the commode, he can then shut the lid to contain odor.

If your loved one is a male, having a urinal to keep beside his bed or chair is a good idea. A urinal is an oblong plastic bottle with an opening at the top large enough for the penis. A man who needs to urinate can simply insert his penis into the opening and "take care of business."

Finally, if bedbound, the person may be able to use a bedpan. Offer the bedpan regularly so that he gets used to using it at certain intervals. This is called bowel and bladder training.

Incontinence Supplies

If your loved one is incontinent all or part of the time, there are many supplies on the market that will make your life as a caregiver much easier.

Panty Liners

Women who experience stress incontinence caused by temporary pressure on the bladder such as laughing, coughing, or sneezing may benefit from wearing panty liners. Panty liners are pads that are attached to the underwear by an adhesive strip. They absorb moisture and odor and protect the skin, but they must be changed if they become fully saturated.

Pull-Ups

Pull-ups are disposable underwear that can be stepped into and out of. They are appropriate for people who can still stand and bear weight, but they do not work well for bedbound seniors.

Adult Diapers (Briefs)

Adult diapers are made of plastic and absorbent materials and are held in place with adhesive tabs. They are especially useful for incontinent persons who are confined to bed.

Absorbent Pads (Chux)

Absorbent pads come in different sizes and can be placed on the seat of a chair or on top of a mattress to protect the surface. When caring for someone who is bedbound, you can avoid a mess by placing a diaper on the person and putting one or two absorbent pads under her to catch any bodily wastes that leak from the diaper.

Changing Pull-Ups

Changing pull-ups is relatively straightforward. Assist your loved one to the bathroom and help him stand up. Encourage him to use handrails to help maintain balance. Never have a senior grab onto a towel rack because these racks are not meant to support the weight of a human and may break or pull away from the wall, causing your loved one to fall. If your loved one has trouble standing, even with the support of handrails, consider using an assisted standing lift to help maintain balance.

Be sure to tell your loved one what you are doing at each step. A confused person may strike out if the caregiver simply starts removing clothes without warning.

When the person is secure on his feet, remove his pants. If they are soiled, set them aside to be washed. Then remove the pull-ups. Pull them down his legs and assist him in stepping out of them, one foot at a time. Place them in plastic bag for disposal.

Next, thoroughly clean the perineal (genital) area with wipes. You can do this task while the person is standing or, if he prefers, while he is sitting on the toilet or commode. Make sure you remove all traces of urine and feces. Then apply lotion as a moisture barrier. Finally, get a fresh pair of pull-ups (and pants, if necessary) and assist your loved one with putting them on.

Changing Diapers

Change diapers as soon as you notice that they are wet or soiled. This will help protect the skin and prevent pressure ulcers from forming. Keeping your loved one as clean as possible is also a dignity issue.

To change the diaper, unfasten the adhesive tabs. Then have the person roll on their side so that they are facing away from you. If they are unable to turn themselves, you can assist them by using a draw sheet—a sheet under the body to help facilitate transfers and repositioning—or by placing your hands on the hips and rolling them away from you. Never try to turn your loved one by the arms or shoulders, as doing so could cause injury.

Remove the diaper and place it in a plastic bag for disposal. Then use wipes to clean your loved one's perineal area. You may have to turn the person onto his back to wipe away feces or urine between the thighs. When the skin is clean, apply lotion as a moisture barrier.

When you finish, the person should again be facing away from you. If the absorbent pad is soiled, roll the pad towards your loved one's body so that the soiled part of the pad is on the inside of the rolled up pad. As you roll the pad, apply gentle traction to pull it from beneath your loved one's body. Then place it in a plastic bag. You may need to change the bed linens if they are also soiled.

Next, take a fresh absorbent pad and roll it in half lengthwise. Place the rolled edge as far under the body as you can. Place an adult diaper with the absorbent surface next to your loved one's bottom. Assist him in rolling over on his back. Fasten the diaper and check to make sure the surface of the diaper is smooth, not creased. Lying on creases can be uncomfortable and can compromise the skin. Next, walk around to the other side of the bed, grasp the rolled-up edge of the absorbent pad, and pull it towards you. By the time you are finished, your loved one should be lying in the middle of the pad. If your loved one is large, you may want to use more than one pad to protect as much of the bedding as possible.

Indwelling Foley Catheters

A catheter is a small tube that is inserted into the urethra to drain urine from the bladder. An indwelling catheter is a catheter that is left in place for the long term. With an indwelling catheter, the tube is held in place in the body by a small balloon that is inflated with saline solution, and the urine drains into a bag that hangs from the frame of the bed or is attached to the leg. Make sure that the drainage bag is always at a lower level than your loved one's bladder (about hip level). If the bag is secured above the bladder, urine will not be able to drain properly.

The Foley catheter is the most common type of indwelling catheter. A doctor might suggest the use of a Foley for several reasons. One is to preserve the skin integrity of a person with incontinence. Having frequent "accidents" can leave the skin in the perineal area raw and ulcerated.

Another reason a doctor might consider a Foley is bladder dysfunction. This occurs when for some reason, such as a spinal injury or an enlarged prostate, the senior is unable to empty his bladder naturally. In these cases, the Foley drains urine that would otherwise build up in the bladder and become toxic.

The Foley catheter has at least two significant risks. One is the risk of infection. Anytime hardware, such as tubing, is introduced into the body, it creates a potential pathway for infection. People with Foley catheters are prone to urinary tract infections. You can minimize this risk with good catheter care. If you notice that your loved one's urine is cloudy, unusually smelly, or red-tinged, report it to the doctor immediately. If your loved one who has a Foley shows signs of increased confusion or agitation, report this as well. Sometimes the only symptoms of urinary tract infections in older adults are behavioral changes.

The other risk that a Foley catheter carries is the risk of injury to the urethra. This most commonly occurs when a confused person pulls the Foley out without deflating the balloon that is holding it in place. If your loved one tugs at the Foley catheter or threatens to remove it, you may have to purchase special clothing, such as pants that fit backwards, that make it harder for your loved one to reach the catheter.

Cleaning the Catheter

The first step in catheter care is keeping the area around the urethra as clean as possible to avoid infection. Cleaning should occur about once every eight hours. Your loved one may be able to clean the catheter area himself, in which case you provide the needed supplies and check when your loved one is finished to make sure that the area really is clean and that there are no signs of infection such as pain, redness, and swelling around the catheter site.

If your loved one requires your assistance to clean the site, use the following supplies: a basin of warm water, soap or soapless cleaner, antiseptic wipes, and gauze pads. Wash your hands and put on gloves.

Explain to your loved one exactly what you are doing with each step of the procedure. Most people become alarmed and even combative when someone attempts to touch their genital area without warning.

Have the person lie on their back in bed. Move any clothing or diapers out of the way so that you can see the catheter. Use the wipes or, if your loved one prefers, soap and water to carefully clean the skin around the catheter. Then use antiseptic wipes or gauze soaked in warm water to clean the catheter tubing. Start where the catheter enters the urethra and wipe down, away from the body. Do not tug too hard on the tubing, or it may become dislodged. When you are finished, make sure the tubing isn't twisted or kinked anywhere. Then help your loved one replace his clothing.

Emptying the Catheter Bag

Another important part of catheter care is emptying the bag that collects the urine. You need to do this whenever you notice it is getting full. Allow your loved one to help with all or part of this process, as able. You will need a container such as a urinal or basin, antiseptic wipes, and plenty of paper towels. Although this procedure should not cause your loved one any pain or embarrassment, it is important to tell him what you are going to do.

Wash your hands and put on gloves. Then place the paper towels below the drainage bag to catch any urine that might splash on the floor. Place the container that will be catching the urine on the paper towels. Next, find the drainage spout on the urine collection bag and open it. Allow the urine to drain into the basin. Close the spout and wipe it clean with sterile wipes. Then flush the urine down the toilet.

If the doctor is concerned about your loved one's urine output, they may ask you to measure it. You can do this by draining the urine into a container with measuring marks, such as a urinal.

Flushing the Catheter

If a catheter becomes clogged, it will need to be flushed or irrigated. If your loved one receives professional care in the home, a nurse may take care of this procedure. If you are doing it yourself, ask the doctor how often you should flush the catheter and which irrigation solution should be used. Your doctor will probably have you purchase a catheter irrigation kit, which contains a catheter syringe and the type of solution your doctor has chosen.

Flushing the catheter is one way that an infection may be introduced into the bladder, so wash your hands and put on gloves before approaching your loved one. As always, explain what you are going to do. It's a good idea to empty the collection bag before flushing the catheter.

Fill the syringe in the kit with the prescribed amount of irrigation solution and set it aside for the moment. Place an absorbent pad on the floor beneath the drainage bag. Find the place where the catheter tubing connects to the drainage bag tubing and swab it clean with an alcohol wipe. Then, pull the Foley catheter tubing and the drainage bag tubing apart. Plug the drainage bag to avoid leaks and set it to one side. Next, insert an empty syringe into the catheter tubing and, depending on what kind of syringe you are using, gently squeeze the bulb at the end of the syringe or pull back on the plunger. This will allow you to clear any urine from the bladder.

Once you have removed all urine from the bladder, remove the syringe from the tubing and place the syringe in a plastic bag for disposal. Next, take the syringe you filled earlier and insert it into the catheter tubing. Using the plunger or the bulb, inject the irrigation solution into the catheter tubing. Don't rush this step, as it might cause an unpleasant sensation of fullness in your loved one's bladder. If you meet with resistance, do not force the fluid in. Instead, follow the directions for reattaching the catheter bag and call your doctor for advice.

Once you have injected the fluid into the tubing, pull back on the plunger so that the fluid re-enters the syringe. Then remove the syringe and place it in a plastic bag for disposal. Clean the catheter tubing with an alcohol wipe. Then pick up the drainage bag, pull the plug, and clean the drainage bag tubing with a wipe. Once these areas are clean, you can reconnect the catheter tubing and the drainage bag.

Removing the Catheter

As long as the catheter is open and running, there is no need to remove the old one and insert a new one. Still, there might come a time when the catheter becomes plugged or malfunctions in some other way. If a catheter needs changing, most doctors will take care of it in the office or will send a nurse out to handle the matter.

If the doctor leaves it up to you, your first step, of course, will be removing the old catheter. Wash your hands, put on gloves, and gather an absorbent pad and a basin to catch bodily fluids. You will also need a small, sharp pair of scissors.

Remember that the catheter is held in place in the bladder by a small balloon inflated with saline solution. The easiest way to deflate this balloon in a Foley catheter is to take a small pair of scissors and cut the balloon port—a small tube spout that forms a "Y" from the main catheter tube. You should see fluid drain out once you have cut the drain port. When all of the fluid has drained, gently pull the catheter out. Stop immediately if you feel any resistance.

If the fluid doesn't drain, it probably means the balloon end of the catheter is blocked. You can try to dissolve the balloon by injecting 10 ml of mineral oil through the inflation port. Wait fifteen minutes. If the fluid still hasn't drained, inject another 10 ml of mineral oil. If that doesn't drain the fluid, do not even try to pull the catheter from the urethra. Instead, call your doctor. Your doctor will probably suggest that your loved one go to the nearest emergency room so that the staff there can finish the job.

Placing a New Catheter

The new catheter and all the supplies you need to insert it will come in a sterile kit. Your doctor will probably provide it, but if not, a kit can be purchased at most pharmacies or medical equipment companies. Kits are not created exactly alike, but they all have the same basic components, which are explained below.

Tear the plastic wrapping from the catheter kit and dispose of it. Wash your hands. Explain to your loved one exactly what you will be doing and why. Advise your loved one that women often feel an uncomfortable pressure during catheter insertion, and men feel what they commonly describe as a "sharp pinch."

If your loved one is female, help her lie on her back and assist her in spreading her legs and raising her knees. Depending on her condition, you may need to help her remain in this position by using positioning pillows.

Place the kit within easy reaching distance—between the legs is a good place—and open it. The first item you will take out of the kit is an absorbent pad, which goes beneath the buttocks to catch any urine or other fluids. The next item is a paper "drape" that goes between the legs and covers the genital area except for the urethra. This helps avoid the spread of infection and enhances the person's privacy.

Next, put on a pair of sterile gloves. Take hold of the catheter tubing and find the balloon port. Inject a small amount of saline solution into the port to make sure that the balloon inflates. If it does not, the kit is defective and you will need to obtain a new one before proceeding.

Open the small package of lubricant and lubricate the end of the tubing that will be inserted into the urethra. This will make the insertion less uncomfortable.

Use the sterile swabs provided in the kit to thoroughly clean the skin around the urethra. Tell your loved one what you will be doing before you touch her and let her know that the sterile swab might feel cold and wet.

When the skin is clean, gently insert the lubricated tubing into the person's urethra. Warn her that she might feel some pressure or feel as if she has to urinate. Watch for urine to appear in the tube. When it does, advance the tubing another 2.5 to 5 centimeters. Then, inject the balloon port with saline solution to hold the catheter in place.

Hang the urine collection bag on the bed frame, making sure it is positioned lower than the hips. As an added precaution against your loved one pulling the catheter out, you may also want to use medical tape to secure the tube against her thigh.

When you are finished inserting the catheter, place all of the disposable equipment in a plastic bag. Help your loved one lower her legs and replace any clothing you may have removed. Cover her with a blanket or a bed cover and help her assume a comfortable position in bed. Tell her that while the catheter is in her bladder, she may feel as if she needs to urinate, but that she doesn't have to worry about having an accident because the catheter is already draining the urine from her bladder.

If you are inserting a catheter in a male, there are only a few differences. The man's legs should be spread at about a 45-degree angle. To clean the area around the urethra, wrap your hand around the man's penis and, beginning in the middle (the urethral opening), swab in ever-increasing circles until you have cleaned the entire glans. You should insert the catheter about six or seven inches. Men are likely to feel more discomfort from the insertion of a catheter than are women.

Stoma or Ostomy Care

Your loved one's illness or injury, such as colon cancer or a wound to the abdomen, may have necessitated removal of part of the intestines. If this is the case, there will be an opening in the abdomen called a stoma, through which feces is eliminated. The feces are collected in a disposable bag that fits over the stoma. Because of the high risk of skin irritation or ulceration, it is important to keep the ostomy bag clean. You will have to clean or replace the ostomy bag whenever feces are eliminated.

You will need a bedpan, an absorbent pad, a bath blanket, a clean ostomy bag and belt (if you will be changing the ostomy), soap or soapless cleaner, a basin of warm water, alcohol wipes, cream or lotion to protect the skin, a couple of towels, and a plastic trash bag. Before providing ostomy care, wash your hands and put on gloves. Tell your loved one what you are going to be doing. Help him lie down on his back in bed. Place an absorbent pad under the body to protect the bed linens. Expose the ostomy site, being careful to keep all other parts of the body covered for privacy and warmth.

Gently remove the ostomy bag. If you are planning to reuse it, place it in the bedpan or a clean basin. If you are discarding it, place it in your plastic bag. If the odor, color, consistency or amount of feces seems unusual, notify your loved one's doctor.

Using soap and water, or an alcohol wipe, carefully wash the area around the stoma, pat dry, and apply any creams or lotions ordered by the doctor. If you are using a clean ostomy bag, place it over the stoma. Make sure the bottom of the bag is clamped. If you are reusing the old bag, put on a new pair of gloves. Empty the old bag into the toilet and wash it using any cleanser and deodorant prescribed by your doctor. Change gloves again, go back to your loved one and apply the newly clean ostomy bag. After you have changed the ostomy bag and provided stoma care, help your loved one dress and get comfortable in or out of bed.

Learning to handle your loved one's toileting needs can be a difficult task for a caregiver. Next to helping with elimination, dressing your loved one is a relatively easy task. The next chapter provides advice on what kind of clothes to buy, how to help your loved one select appropriate clothing to wear each day, and how to help your loved one get into, and out of clothing.

THIRTEEN

How to Dress

From your point of view, it would probably be easier to keep your loved one in a hospital gown or nightgown all day. Just think how easy it would be to provide care if all you needed to do was change a gown from time to time. Unless your loved one is bedbound and requires extensive physical care, however, it's usually not a good idea to keep him in a gown all the time. Getting dressed and cleaned up in the morning can get a day off to a positive start. Have you ever had a day when you started out dragging but felt better after showering and putting on your favorite suit? The same thing can happen for home bound seniors.

Clothes are important because they are a part of our identity. Even as adults, most of us can probably remember spending a few too many hours shopping for the perfect dress for a party or a leisure suit to take on a vacation. Your loved one, too, wants to feel good about his or her clothes and identity.

Personal Preference vs. Practicality

If you want to order clothes that are tailored to your loved one's specific needs, you can do so on several websites. Two of the more popular ones include Buck and Buck (http://www.buckandbuck.com/patient_clothing.shtml) and Clothing Solutions (http://www.clothingsolutions.com/).

If the senior can get out of bed for any period of time, it enhances self-esteem to wear street clothes during the times that they are up. If your loved one is capable of making choices, allow him or her to select the clothes to wear each day. If it is overwhelming because there are too many options, or the clothing choice is inappropriate due to the weather or some other factor, try selecting two or three appropriate outfits and allowing them to choose between them. Unless there is strenuous objection, make sure the wardrobe consists of clothes that are comfortable, attractive, and easy to put on and remove. Adaptive clothing often features Velcro strips or snaps which can be easier to manage than tiny zippers or buttons. As a loved one's disease progresses, they may gain or lose weight. Make sure that clothes fit properly and buy new ones if the ones they are currently wearing become too loose or too tight.

People who have dementia may be physically capable of dressing themselves but may not be able to remember how to do so. If this is the case with your loved one, provide verbal and tactile cues. Keep your instructions brief and to the point and only give one instruction at a time. For instance, you might touch his hand lightly and say, "Put this arm through the sleeve." There may also come a time when an older adult is mostly or totally dependent on you to assist with dressing.

Undressing

As always, tell your loved one what you are going to do and provide as much privacy as possible. When undressing your loved one, start at the top and work down. To remove a garment that fits over the head, like a nightgown, undo any fasteners. This may require you to assist in rolling them onto the side away from you. Gather the shirt or nightgown around the neck. If your loved is weaker on one side than the other, remove clothing from the strongest arm first by gently sliding the arm down the sleeve. Be careful not to twist the arm or allow the fabric to catch on dry flesh and cause skin tears. Once they are free of the item of clothing, lift the garment over the head. Again, be careful not to pull the hair or damage the skin on the face.

If your loved one is wearing trousers, shorts, or underpants that need to be removed, undo the fasteners. If the person can stand or raise the buttocks in bed enough for you to slide the clothing down, assist to do so. If the person cannot stand or lift the buttocks, help them roll to the strong side first and ease the pants down on the weaker side. Then help him roll to the weak side and pull the pants down on the other side. Help roll him onto his back and slide the pants down the legs.

Dressing

If your loved one wears adult diapers, you need not worry about underpants. If they wear pull-ups or regular underwear, have them sit on the side of the bed or lie on their back if they are unable to sit up. Gently work one leg into the underpants and then the other. Slide the underpants up the legs as far as you can. Then assist them in standing or ask them to lift the buttocks so that you can slide the underpants up the rest of the way. If they cannot lift the buttocks, help to roll them onto the stronger side and pull the underpants up their weaker side. Then help roll them to their weaker side and pull the underpants up on the stronger side. Position your loved one on their back and make sure the underpants fit comfortably.

If the person you are caring for is a woman, she may choose to wear a bra. To help her put it on, slide each arm through the appropriate bra strap so that the front of the bra covers her breasts. Then help her sit up or turn to the side facing away from you so that you can fasten the bra at the back. Help position her on her back again and make sure that the bra fits comfortably over each breast and that none of the straps are twisted. A woman who can still help dress herself may prefer to wear a bra that fastens in front.

Some women would rather wear undershirts than bras. Assist with an undershirt by gathering the top and bottom together at the neck opening and slipping the garment over the head. As always, be sure to let her know what you are going to do first so she does not become frightened or anxious. Starting with the weak side first, slide the arms through the sleeves of the undershirt, pull it down, and smooth out any wrinkles.

Pants or short

Gather the top and the bottom of the garment and work the legs through the openings one at a time. Pull them up as you did with the underpants and fasten any buttons, zippers, or snaps.

Pullovers

Putting on a garment that goes over the head is exactly like putting on an undershirt. Start with the weak side first and proceed gently to avoid twisting the arm into a painful position or inflicting a skin tear.

Tops that fasten in front

As always, start with the weakest side. Stand facing them and place your own hand and arm through the wristband of the shirt. Gently take your loved one's hand and slide the garment from your arm onto theirs. Adjust the sleeve at the shoulder. Help them sit up or lean forward and bring the top around the back.

Then guide the strong arm into the sleeve and adjust at the shoulder. Finish by fastening any snaps, zippers, or buttons.

Tops that fasten in back

As with tops that fasten in front, start with the weakest side, place the sleeve over your own arm, take your loved one's hand, and gently slide the sleeve from your arm to theirs. Adjust at the shoulder. Use the same procedure for the sleeve on the other side. Help them sit up or lean forward, bring the sides of the shirt around to the back, and fasten it in place.

Socks

Gather the sock in your hand so that the toe and the opening are close together. Ease the sock onto the person's foot, making sure to position the heel of the sock and any seams correctly. Pull the sock up the leg.

Shoes

Choose shoes with non-skid soles. Women should avoid high heels due to the risk of falling. Shoes should fit comfortably, neither too loosely nor too tightly. Put your loved one's shoes on by loosening any shoelaces or fastenings and easing the shoe onto your loved one's foot. A shoe horn may help the heel slide into the shoe more easily. Make sure you have the correct shoe on the correct foot, since wearing shoes backwards can be uncomfortable and can cause sore places on the feet. Fasten the shoe securely but not too tightly.

The simple act of getting dressed, even with assistance, gives your loved one a chance to stretch her muscles and move around a little. The next chapter discusses more formal types of exercise from which an older adult may benefit.

Isabelle's Story

Isabelle La, West Coast Regional Director of Home Care Assistance, recounts her experiences with a charming couple who had been married for 65 years. She met Pat in a rehab facility, where she was recovering after falling and fracturing her pelvic bone. Sam had been urging the rehab staff every day to release his sweetheart back home so she could get out of the hospital gown and back to her own clothes, her own life, and her own routine. The orders finally came through to have Pat return home with live-in caregivers.

Sam was eager to get Pat back home and back to who she was. He somehow felt that once she was back in her own home, she'd be back to normal. In her own clothes and in her home environment, Sam was sure Pat would be more comfortable with who she was and what her place in the world was as Sam's sweetheart.

Sam and Pat had been together as long as they could remember, high school sweethearts that continued to love each other well into their 90s. Sam had his own successful business near their home, driving back and forth even at the ripe old age of 91, and Pat's routine as a housewife would always be to have meals prepared for breakfast, lunch and dinner since Sam would come home to greet his wife during meals each day. Sam would dress in his work clothes each morning, comprised of a tucked in, collared shirt and khaki slacks, held together with a belt. He liked giving the appearance of a well-put-together boss that was hard-working but approachable. That was who he was and he chose to express that in how he wore clothes every day at work. Pat lived for Sam and when he came back every day, she'd be dressed up for him, waiting with a smile and her cute sweaters and nice pants.

When Pat started showing signs of forgetfulness and then was ultimately diagnosed with dementia, Sam was very upset. They had been living independently into their late 80s and Sam refused to accept that he needed any help taking care of Pat. He would dress her, go to work in his usual way and when he came back for lunch of dinner, meals were no longer waiting for him. He would find Pat dressed in the same clothes he left her in, sometimes soiled or half off. When Pat fell and broke her pelvic bone and wasn't allowed to be released from the rehab facility until live-in caregiving was arranged, that was Sam's first time admitting and allowing any help into his life.

The live-in caregiver, Anita, was the bright light at the end of their tunnel. Having worked in home care as long as she did, she knew how she could help Sam and Pat regain what they were seeking. What they wanted was a way back into their old habits, despite some of the changes that had been occurring with Pat's mobility and mental state. Anita made it a point to get Pat dressed and cleaned every morning, even though Pat began to get resistant to showers. Anita found a closet full of clothes that had hardly been touched for some time and took them all out for Pat to wear. She even suggested some modifications for the clothing so that Pat would not have as much trouble putting them on, like adding Velcro snaps instead of buttons or having the same style of pants in an elastic waist instead of a zipper and button waist. She would dress Pat in her favorite sweaters and pants every day for breakfast and made sure that Pat and breakfast were both at the table before Sam left for work in the mornings. During lunch, before Sam came home, Anita made sure Pat's sweaters and pants from the morning were still clean and, if not, she would change her shirt or remove some stains so that Pat always looked her best for Sam, like she used to. Anita did the same thing for dinner and, before we knew it, Sam was overjoyed at having his wife back. It was as simple as having her in the proper clothes within the usual times of day to make Sam and Pat feel that they were getting back something they had lost.

This continued for two more years but, unfortunately and surprisingly, Sam passed away in his sleep at the age of 93. Even with Pat's dementia, Anita knew there was a change – she would turn around every time the door opened and yell out for "Sam, Sam, Sam?" but it would never be Sam. However, Anita continues to dress Pat up during meal times and, somehow, Anita thinks this whole process of getting her dressed for the day and making Pat look her best really helps Pat get through a time where she is still expecting Sam to come back home for a meal. Meanwhile, Pat is still in her pretty sweaters and pants, waiting for Sam as she always did and, until his last day, Sam had come home to the Pat he knew when they first fell in love.

This story illustrates how clothes can be a part of how we identify with others and ourselves. Sam felt Pat was being wel-cared for because she was always so properly dressed in the clothes she had worn before her fall and dementia, which was a comfort for him. Though we won't know how Pat feels about her clothes, her caregiver, Anita, explained that even though it is a bit of a struggle to get Pat to shower and get dressed, when she is seated at the table for her meals, she channels an inner peace.

The next chapter focuses on exercise for seniors and how to do simple movements in a safe and beneficial fashion.

FOURTEEN

How To Exercise Safely

Doctors recommend that healthy adults should engage in at least 30 minutes per day of moderate to intense physical activity. Although seniors typically have physical deficits, they too should remain as active as physically possible. That's because muscles that go unused atrophy and contract over time. Once contractures begin to occur, it is almost impossible to regain lost mobility. So this chapter looks at different types of physical activities that older adults may be able to engage in.

Activities of Daily Living (ADLs)

People who are frail or non-ambulatory often find that simple ADLs such as getting dressed, eating, and transferring from bed to wheelchair are enough to give them a challenging workout. Completing ADLs may be considered an important form of exercise. Always encourage older adults to do as much possible, even if that means an activity will take longer. For instance, it takes much less time to simply dress or feed a person with Alzheimer's disease than it does to provide the verbal and physical cues necessary to dress or feed themselves. If you perform the activity for a person, however, you have denied them a chance to engage in healthy movement.

Sometimes seniors get used to being waited on by caregivers. During the early days of your loved one's illness, you may be tempted to do too much out of sympathy. If your loved one refuses to perform tasks of which they are physically capable, be understanding, but firm. Don't simply withdraw your assistance, but encourage your loved one to take a little more personal responsibility for their own care. Instead of brushing his hair, for instance, you might hand over the brush and say, "I need to get a load of laundry started, so I'll let you brush your hair this morning."

These changes will take a little getting used to for both of you, but they are a good start to engaging your loved one in physical activity.

Instrumental Activities of Daily Living (IADLs)

IADLs are activities that people perform in order to live independently. Examples include cleaning the house, feeding the pets, preparing meals, grocery shopping, and managing a budget. If your loved one is capable of engaging in some of the physical IADLs, like preparing a simple meal under your supervision or dusting the living room, encourage them to do so. Even something as simple as polishing silverware or folding laundry provides exercise for the hands, arms, and fingers. Another IADL your loved one may be able to perform with you is shopping. Rather than having them use a store-provided scooter, try having them push a shopping cart around the store to give their legs some exercise. Shopping can also be a workout for the mind. Ask your loved one to help you spot the items you need on the store shelves.

Walking

Keep your loved one ambulatory for as long as possible. Just walking around the house or the yard a few times is better than simply sitting in a wheelchair. Many older adults have a "transfer" wheelchair that they use when they go out, but walk around the house with the assistance of a cane or walker.

Stationary Bike Pedal Exerciser

A stationary bike pedal exerciser consists of a stand that supports two bike pedals. Your loved one can sit on the edge of the bed or on a wheelchair to use the exerciser, which provides a great workout for the legs and helps keep the joints in the knees loose. A stationary bike pedal exerciser can be ordered online for a little over a hundred dollars. You may also be able to purchase one at a pharmacy or a medical equipment store.

Maura Barilaro, RN, Director of Nursing for Home Care Assistance, Washington, DC, helped a client with a unique approach to maintaining physical activity.

This particular client had a condition known as cerebellum atrophy, which caused her to become wheelchair dependent and non-ambulatory. The live-in caregiver assigned to this client put her feet in the pedal bike exerciser and moved her feet so that she maintained muscle mass and slowed the process of atrophy to her lower extremities. The client jokes that it is "the bike that goes nowhere."

The live-in caregiver also puts the bike exerciser on the tray table and sits the client in front of it. The aide then encourages her to move the pedal of the bike with her arms. Despite the cerebellum atrophy, this woman still had full range of motion in her upper extremities.

Ball/Balloon Play

Ball and balloon play consists of encouraging your loved one to hit or kick a beach ball or a balloon. Alternatively, you can ask your loved one to catch the balloon and throw it back to you.

This form of exercise encourages movement of both the arms and legs and can be a lot of fun. However, it isn't for everyone. Seniors with dementia might be startled to have a ball or balloon tossed in their direction, and some feel as if this activity is too childlike.

Judy remembers trying to engage her mother, Margaret, who was in the later stages of dementia, in play with a balloon. At the time, Margaret rarely spoke anymore. She usually just glared when Judy got the balloon out and started tossing it in her direction. One day, Margaret had had enough. She caught the balloon in both hands hard enough to pop it, looked her daughter in the eye, and said, "Don't throw that thing in my face one more time." Judy didn't.

Tai Chi

For seniors troubled by arthritis, limited mobility, or poor balance, Tai Chi could be the perfect exercise. It provides a low impact workout that stretches the muscles and helps improve balance and agility. Some geriatric specialists report that older adults who practice Tai Chi seem to have fewer falls and seem to maintain their mobility longer.

Tai Chi is a workout that you and your loved one can do together. There are several DVDs for beginners on the market and one DVD that is specific to seniors (Tai Chi Exercises for Seniors). If your loved one cannot do all of the exercises shown on the video, have him "sit out" the ones he is not comfortable with and participate in the ones he feels he can safely accomplish.

Range of Motion

The most common form of physician-prescribed exercise for people with severely restricted mobility is called range of motion (ROM). Jennifer Serafin explains: "Basically, you take each joint in the [arms], hands, legs, feet, and fingers, and put it gently through its range of motion or movement comfort zone." Serafin warns caregivers to talk with their loved one's doctor or physical therapist prior to attempting ROM. In some cases you may wish to have a professional teach you how to do ROM exercises properly, so as not to injure your loved one or yourself. There are two types of ROM: active and passive:

Active ROM

In active ROM, your loved one moves most or all of their own limbs, while you provide verbal cues ("Point your toes towards the ceiling") and minor physical assistance. You verbally encourage active participation from your loved one as much as possible. Even if they are paralyzed on one side of their body, for instance, they can still move the other side.

Passive ROM

Passive ROM means that you extend and flex your loved one's muscles with little or no assistance. For instance, passive ROM may be used if a person is unconscious, quadriplegic, or too confused to follow verbal and tactile cues.

The next chapter takes a look at a private duty agency called Home Care Assistance and explains how this agency uses its unique training philosophy to produce talented, skilled, and compassionate caregivers.

FIFTEEN

The Home Care Assistance Approach

Home Care Assistance agencies are located throughout the United States, Canada, and Puerto Rico. They provide professional caregivers to assist clients with activities of daily living and instrumental activities of daily living. Caregivers can be hired for a minimum of a few hours to a maximum of 24/7 care. No long-term contracts are required. They can function as an individual's primary caregiver, or they can provide respite so the person providing the lion's share of the care can take a break.

One specialty of Home Care Assistance is providing live-in care. Studies suggest that more than 89% of seniors express a preference for remaining at home rather than going to a facility. Home Care Assistance is an agency that can help you honor these wishes.

Balanced Care

Balanced Care, the method Home Care Assistance uses to train all of its caregiver employees, was developed through the study of extremely long-lived elders in the Okinawa region of Japan. The method attempts to tap into elements of these elders' lifestyles that extend life and health.

Based on research and observation, the two most important factors in living a long, full life appear to be moderation and variety. The Balanced Care Method™ applies these principles to several aspects of home care.

The diet promoted by the Balanced Care Method is rich in variety and places special emphasis on vegetables, fruits, whole grains, lean proteins, flavonoids, and Omega-3 rich foods.

Because people remain healthier when they engage in physical activity, Home Care Assistance caregivers are trained to teach clients low-impact exercises like methodically stretching all of the muscle groups.

Home Care Assistance caregivers learn that they should do more than just meet a client's basic physical needs. They should also encourage socialization through phone calls, letters, emails, and, if the client is able, outings to favorite activities and events. Home Care Assistance employees are also expected to spend at least an hour each day conversing or otherwise interacting with the client.

Respect is another issue addressed by training. All too often, seniors or people suffering from a disabling condition that renders them home bound are addressed very informally by paid caregivers. ("Let me help you with that, Grandma." "Are you hungry, sweetie?") Home Care Assistance caregivers are trained to treat all clients with respect by asking them on the initial visit how they would like to be addressed and then following the client's wishes. As a further show of respect to the client, caregivers are expected to maintain acceptable hygiene and a professional appearance at all times.

Caregivers are taught that a live-in client may find it embarrassing to accept help with personal care from a stranger. They learn many methods for putting clients at ease. For instance, caregivers learn to allow the client to do as much for themselves as is possible. If a client does need assistance, the caregiver provides it in a gentle, matter-of-fact manner, using proper names for body parts and explaining what he is going to do before they do it.

Home Care Assistance caregivers never make reference to the personal care they have provided after the care is completed. To further protect dignity and privacy, the caregiver never discusses the care with a third party. Finally, all caregivers are instructed to hold all information about their clients in the strictest confidence. The client's personal, medical, and financial information is never shared with anyone outside the agency.

Careful screening procedures and training in the Balanced Care Method produces competent, compassionate, and effective caregivers who know how best to help the home care patient.

If you would like to contact Home Care Assistance to see if there is an agency in your area or to discuss your loved one's care, you can reach them through their website at **http://www.homecareassistance.com** or via email at **info@homecareassistance.com**. You can also send a letter to corporate headquarters at Home Care Assistance, 148 Hawthorne Avenue, Palo Alto, CA 94301.